# Aluminum Detox

# An Easy Solution

# Dr. Bill McGraw

`The information found in this book is for educational and research purposes and should not substitute for professional naturopathic services in the event of serious disease

Copyright © 2021 Dr. Bill McGraw

www.newaquatechpanama.com

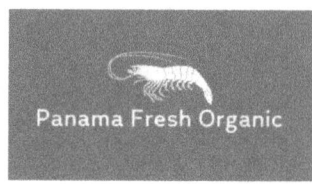

"growing clean, mercury-free seafood"

All rights reserved. No part of this book may be reproduced, stored in a retrieval system, or transmitted by any means, electronic, mechanical, photocopying, recording, or otherwise, without written permission from the author

Editing, formatting, cover design etc. by Dr. Bill McGraw

10 9 8 7 6 5 4 3 2 1

*This book is dedicated to my sweet, darling wife Gladys and my dearest sister Noreen for their support and encouragement, making this book possible*

# Contents

**Chapter 1. Aluminum, An Introduction** ............................ 1

**Chapter 2. Aluminum Production and the Environment.** 11

    Fluoride in Our Drinking Water .................. 14

    The Ocean and the Apex Predators................ 16

    Freshwater.................................................. 17

    Silica and Oxalate, Two Aluminum Chelators for Plants ................................................................. 18

    Aquatic Animals ........................................ 21

    Oxalates and Toxicity in Humans................ 22

    Aluminum Toxicity in Bees ......................... 25

    In the Air .................................................. 25

    Aluminum Absorbed Through the Nose and Lungs ... 28

**Chapter 3. Sources of Aluminum Toxicity** ...................... 31

    Aluminum in Water and Drinks ................... 31

    Aluminum in Food ..................................... 33

Aluminum in Antiperspirants ............................................. 38

    Aluminum in Medicine ................................................ 40

    Aluminum in Vaccines ................................................ 42

**Chapter 4. Aluminum and Disease ........................................ 47**

    Aluminum, The Universal Metabolic Disruptor ......... 47

    Alzheimer's and Other Neuro Degenerative Disease. 48

    Cardiovascular Disease ................................................ 53

    Cell Longevity, Osteoporosis and Hip Fractures ......... 54

**Chapter 5. Measuring Aluminum in the Human Body .... 57**

**Chapter 6. Aluminum Detox, It's in The Water ............... 59**

    The Blue Zones, More Irrefutable Proof ..................... 65

**Chapter 7. OSA in the Diet and Other Detox Methods .. 69**

    Ionic Foot Baths .......................................................... 75

    Glutathione, The Chelator the Body Makes ............... 76

**Chapter 8. Conclusion, Depopulation and the End Gam. 79**

Sources and Further Reading ........................................... 84

Index .................................................................................. 92

# Chapter 1

## Aluminum, An Introduction

What do you think of when you hear the word aluminum? Most people would think aluminum cans, maybe cookware, aluminum foil, ladders maybe even aluminum siding on your house. But these common things are a small and minor part of the real story behind aluminum and why it is so important. Notably in today's headlines of major, fake media news, you would never hear anything about aluminum used as an adjuvant. An adjuvant is supposed to work together with the components of a vaccine to create an immunity against an infectious agent. Yet, as you will read here, aluminum used as an adjuvant causes more harm than good and vaccines that don't contain aluminum invoke an entirely separate immune response pathway compared to aluminum containing vaccines. Attenuated viruses and bacteria, without heavy metal adjuvants, actually create proper immunity against infection. So why is aluminum even used? Well, this is no time to be naïve or ignorant so we will engage the answers that are far beyond probable and further than those considered most likely, the answers that are obtained from a long trip down the rabbit hole that ends. All rabbit holes eventually end. Luckily, you don't have to find your way back. The end is the end and the start of a new beginning, an enlightenment. For truth shall set you free, but it will also bind you. Once you know, you cannot unknow. There is only one way forward. Knowledge is still power and power brings freedom. So empower yourself so that you can live free.

This book is filled with facts and few opinions. One out of three elderly people will die of Alzheimer's disease. Within 20 years, one out of every two people will die of Alzheimer's or a similar neuro degenerative disease. This is in the midst of an ever-increasing budget provided to the medical meatheads to find a cure for this incredibly debilitating and damaging disease. Heavy metal toxicity causes Alzheimer's, Parkinson's, multiple sclerosis, amyotrophic lateral sclerosis and dementia. Now if this is the case, as it is overwhelmingly evident in the scientific literature, why does the medical industry not engage in detoxification procedures that remove heavy metals and cure the disease? The truth is to get an MD you are trained for two things in order to cure people from chronic disease: surgery and prescription drugs. For trauma care, the medical industry does an outstanding job, but for chronic disease, patients suffer horribly. There are no classes on nutrition or heavy metal toxicology given to MDs to obtain their degree and well the rest is another hole in the ground (read the book, *World Without Cancer* by G. Edward Griffin).

Well friends, unless you are very young and you are untested and untried, you might reject the truth initially as I have done many times myself, wandering around blind and lost. But once you get a taste of what is real and actual, you will crave for more, but if you never get your first taste, you will never know how sweet and irresistible it is. Thus, we have entered the age of the dichotomy: them and us. People that have been vaccinated and those that have not. People that know the truth and seek it regularly and those that have their head in their behinds. Maybe because the ignorant cannot stand the reality of the truth or they prefer to remain ignorant, or maybe they are genetically and environmentally predisposed to it. Many people told me they took the vaccine because they just want to travel and I think most took it due to fear, promoted by the major media (think 1984, Alexa are vaccines safe? "yes Winston, vaccines are safe and effective, you can trust vaccines they are the cure for all diseases...."). Yeh right, I never liked that black box that my friend has, too damn creepy.

So, the next question you may ponder in this interesting discourse is: why haven't we always had this problem of aluminum toxicity and aluminum causing disease? Well, that is another easy question to answer. Aluminum has existed for many millennia as an unreactive ore stuck many meters below the ground. In the environment with a normal pH above 5.0, aluminum ions exist at a very small fraction, however, when the pH of water or soil drops below 4.7 as in the case of acid rain, like what has happened in the northeastern area of the US, aluminum is released from being bound in rock and clay which then results in mortality to aquatic wildlife at a very low value of just 1.5 parts per million (ppm or mg/L). But aside from acid rain, created from the burning of coal without pollution control devices, pure aluminum became available in the late 1800s with the discovery of the process to create aluminum from ore, and aluminum production has increased to such a status as it can be put into nearly anything and still be cost effective at nearly every level. This includes air, water, food, medicine, vaccines, antiperspirants, food packaging and e-cigarettes. This is very detrimental, as mammals on this planet have evolved without the interference of aluminum, this is the biggest reason why aluminum is so very toxic in small amounts.

Once you know what can kill you, you will live a longer and more pain free life. Maybe we should ask the blue zoners…we will get to talking about them soon enough. Aluminum is incredibly toxic and it is found in many things you would not realize. From the use of aluminum sulfate in water treatment as a way to remove particles in order to make tap water "ok" to drink, to aluminum compounds added to powders to prevent caking as is the case of baking powder, dried milk and pancake mixes.

Aluminum is cheap and it has found a way into many things you would never think would contain it. Did you know that the application of most popular sunscreens will put 200 mg (milligrams) of aluminum in contact with your skin? Even though a minor percentage makes it through your skin, keep in mind that 1.5 parts per million (ppm,

## Aluminum Detox, An Introduction

mg/L or milligrams per liter) of aluminum in water is enough to kill fish. The limit placed on allowable aluminum in drinking water is 0.1 ppm (parts per million). Hard to believe but the regular drinking of water that contains 0.1 ppm aluminum has been scientifically documented to be associated with Alzheimer's disease.

How about deodorants containing antiperspirants that have aluminum? There are over a billion people that use them every day and the industry is worth $80 billion. Antiperspirants contain aluminum chlorohydrate which blocks the release of sweat from underarm sweat glands. This sweat reducing chemical is a contributor to aluminum toxicity. But did you know there are alternatives available that work just as well and are completely free of aluminum? Well why do people continually use aluminum antiperspirants still? The answer can be found in greed, ignorance, complacency and maybe something more sinister. Some people just don't realize how toxic aluminum can be. But you thought that aluminum is safe and effective right? Well, they said the same thing about mercury in amalgam fillings, and now no one in their right mind who has found out about that rabbit coming out of the hole ever questions it. Here in Panama, all dentists are using ceramic or some sort of plastic filling that is 1000 times less toxic. If you ask any young person today about mercury amalgam for use in filling cavities you will likely get a blank stare, but when I was 20 years old, everyone had them. Times change and eventually people get smarter, but on the horizon there is always something new that needs examination. When people get sick, a certain number will go out of their way to find out why, a certain number will venture down the hole made by the rabbit, and most of the time it is through necessity.

I would not be writing this second book on heavy metals if a doctor, any doctor, MD, PhD, ND etc., had found a way to cure my insomnia when I first experienced it 15 years ago. I went to 10 doctors over 10 years before I just figured it out and cured myself. I had mineral deficiencies, in particular, potassium and magnesium, which were caused by mercury toxicity. This was born out by a hair test which showed all three of these variables as important. The hair test showed the minerals that were too high and too low in concentration as described by Dr. Andrew Cutler about 35 years ago in his book about amalgam Illness. Since then, I have taken supplements to cure the deficiency and I have removed enough mercury out of my body to cure the problem. The good news I can provide here is that aluminum is easier to take out of the body, the bad news is that 85% of all aluminum taken into the body can be stored in the brain according to all the peer-reviewed, scientific studies I have read. Hello Alzheimer's.

We will engage in overwhelming proof that aluminum causes Alzheimer's. But the hole has many more twists and turns than that. Part of the problem is major media has a hold of most of the attention of people looking for answers, and their propaganda and disinformation

## Aluminum Detox, An Introduction

campaign is legend. What doesn't kill you only makes you stronger, but if we don't find out how to get the truth out there so people can use it, ignorance is going to result in massive, yet avoidable death (Hi Georgia Guidestones, Agenda 21/30 and the new world order etc.).

What else? I have good friends that have retired out of the military that tell me that chemtrails don't exist and I know they only do that to keep their pensions flowing and maintain their promises. Look, I get that. But it does not change the fact that there are tens of millions of people that can verify the existence of chemtrails and many can provide physical proof. I will discuss the whole chemtrail thing objectively, and you can decide for yourself if that trail is one you want to keep walking on, or down as they say. Chemtrails contain aluminum.

But there is a more detrimental source of aluminum. I know that very few people use aluminum pots and pans anymore, except maybe indigenous people that like the fact that aluminum is easy to work with because it has a low melting point. But this next source is just insane. One out of three people in the modern world suffers from acid reflux, which is the result of mineral deficiencies according to the alternative medicine well-knowns that I listen to regularly. About 25% of those 100s of millions, regularly use aluminum containing antacids that come in handy: sweet flavored colorful tablets that are readily available over the counter. Well, what if I told you that most of those people who take those sweet chewables are going to develop Alzheimer's type diseases if they use too many for too long. But hey! Don't take my word for it, read the warning label that is on the outside of every package. They openly admit it. No I am not kidding.

The biggest part of this story is about water. Aluminum is found in tap water because aluminum sulfate is used to remove particles and make the water "ok" to drink. Approximately 50% of all tap water in the US contains at least 0.1 ppm aluminum and this amount in drinking water has been routinely associated in clinical studies with developing Alzheimer's. However, aluminum in water can be removed with carbon filters and ion exchange resins.

Because we grow food on acid soils and aluminum is raining down in abundance in places like California, our food contains aluminum. But, there is good news, plants are smarter than we are. Plants accumulate silica in their tissues in the form of orthosilicic acid that chelates or removes minor amounts of aluminum as a rock or phytolith that can be found in their tissues. When we eat this phytolith in plants we receive the benefit of aluminum binding in our intestines as well as the orthosilicic acid (OSA) that the plants contain. This OSA is the easy solution I refer to in the title of this book. This is the easy way to get rid of aluminum from your brain, I will describe this process and proof of validity, in great detail. Certain mineral waters contain OSA in good abundance as well and the regular, continual consumption of these waters can reduce the symptoms of Alzheimer's in a matter of months. You can also make a cheaper synthetic mineral water from filtered tap water and simple compounds. Since water cannot be patented, this cure will be kept secret for as long as the darkside can possibly do it. But yet again, don't take my word for it, read all the sources at the end of this book and prove it for yourself.

The medical monopoly described in *World Without Cancer* is only interested in abating the symptoms of most disease and they will tell you that Alzheimer's is a result of old age and it has no cause or cure (no I am not kidding here, look it up). But how is it that so many people live to the age of over 100 in the blue zone? There in the blue zone is where our rabbit hole likely ends. Where water coming out of the ground contains high levels of OSA which binds the aluminum impurities found nearly everywhere and the proof is irrefutable, undeniable and incredibly ignored. I imagine the old folks there don't consider how lucky they are, letting water be their medicine and experiencing an 80% reduction in many chronic diseases. Well at least there, ignorance is bliss. I guess as they say, they are living the dream, and not even knowing it. Nice.

# Chapter 2

## Aluminum Production and the Environment

Aluminum has many properties which make it great to use, such as the fact that it doesn't rust. It is soft, non-magnetic and malleable. Aluminum is the third most abundant element in the earth's crust, however it is permanently bound to other elements and it does not exist as a separate element normally found in nature or in the human body that has not been exposed to some of the many man-made sources of aluminum in air, water, food, medicine, vaccines, e-cigarettes, deodorants, cookware, food and drink containers and sunscreen. Aluminum is naturally bound to the two other most common elements in the earth's crust, silica and oxygen. Together these three elements form over 1000 mineral compounds, all tightly bound together. Aluminum can only be released from these mineral compounds once it is exposed to man-made strong acids or bases such as acid rain formed from sulfur pollution in the atmosphere or from sodium hydroxide used during the aluminum extraction process to form aluminum hydroxide. Pure aluminum is created from a separate, more complicated process in order to obtain pure aluminum for industry.

# Aluminum Detox

When writing my book on mercury toxicity I wondered where it all began. How did so much mercury find its way into the environment? Well, I need to know the same for aluminum. Our story begins in the 1880s, when about the same time many gold miners were calling it quits in California as was indicated by the large decrease in the measured mercury in the atmosphere, a process was developed on the other side of the United States to remove aluminum from the mineral ore that is found in the ground. The process invented came to be known as the Bayer process and it begins by mixing ground-up aluminum ore with hot sodium hydroxide and then the mixture is digested and heated to purify the end-product which is alumina or aluminum hydroxide. By 1886, the Hall-Herold process was developed which allowed the purification of the aluminum element from alumina so that pure aluminum could be used for industrial and chemical applications.

Aluminum would go on to be the most widely used metal across the planet since the discovery of iron during prehistoric times. Aluminum would gain great importance during World Wars 1 and 2 as it was widely used in airplanes and by 1954 it became the most widely used non-ferrous metal, replacing copper (Figure 1.)

Worldwide aluminum production increased by a factor of three times between 1975 and 2005 and it was during this time that the increase can readily be seen in the graph

# Aluminum Production and the Environment

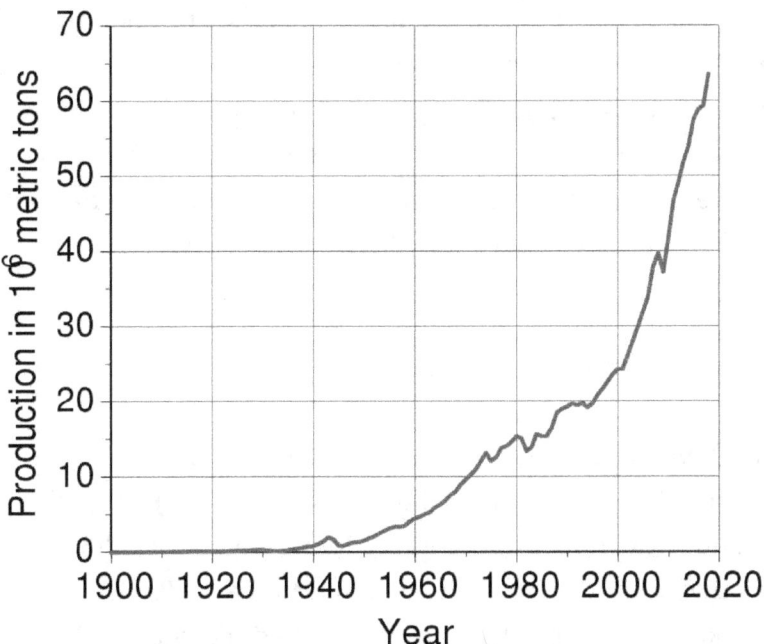

Figure 1. Aluminum production since 1900 in million metric tons (Wikipedia, https://en.wikipedia.org/wiki/Aluminium)

above. The country with the largest increase during this time was of course China. However, Brazil is currently a world leading producer of aluminum and alumina with over 18 million tons cranked out each year. This is because the rainforests there have the highest aluminum content of mineral ores in the world.

Unfortunately, the process to produce pure aluminum requires lots of water and the gross looking wastewater leftover has a pH of 14 and it is incredibly toxic to all life and cannot be used for anything, so it sits in lined ponds and waits to escape, accidentally of course, to flood the environment with toxic heavy metals including an incredibly high concentration of aluminum. The aluminum mining industry produces 150 million metric tons of this waste every year. In addition to this, once mined areas are replanted, they never return to their pristine rainforest conditions.

**Fluoride in Our Drinking Water**

Another twisted part of this tale involves the use of calcium fluoride (or other fluoride compounds) needed to produce the pure aluminum. A fluoride waste product is produced that ends up as sodium fluoride added to drinking water. The first time this was done was in 1945 in Michigan (US), in an attempt to decrease dental cavities in those drinking it. This process continues today as 99.8% of all drinking water in the US contains at least 2 mg/L (milligrams per liter) of fluoride with much of it coming from the making of phosphate fertilizers, again resulting in a fluoride waste product that needed to find a use. The US Public Health Service recommended in 2015 that fluoride content in drinking water should be reduced to 0.7 ppm (parts per million) while the WHO recommends 1.5 (to prevent fluorosis) and the EPA, 4 ppm.

Fluoride in drinking water has been very well documented to cause fluorosis, which is a discoloration and damage to the enamel of teeth. The addition of fluoride waste products created from the aluminum industry added to drinking water has been banned by most countries except for a few in the UK and of course the US, as psychopaths are running (ruining) much of our country. The use of fluoride in drinking water has also been determined to cause skeletal fluorosis which is the process where bones become brittle and tendons and ligaments become calcified. Right now (2021), worldwide hip fractures total 1.7 million per year and this is expected to increase to 6.3 million by 2050. The standard medical response is to replace hip bones with metal implants instead of eliminating the fluoride in the drinking water and fixing the mineral deficiencies which cause fragile bones in the first place. This is classic band aid approach taken by the medical industry in the US. A few medical meatheads suggest ingesting more calcium by itself to solve the problem, which adds to atherosclerosis as excess calcium in the blood is part of the plaque formed which patches damaged arteries caused by inflammation. It takes 10 different elements, including silica, to make bone tissue, so a better option is to supplement with ionic trace minerals or colloidal minerals. It is important to note that people below the age of 50 don't really have hip fractures as they still have enough minerals in their bones. Another important fact is that hip fractures were not common before 1980 compared to what they are today.

**The Ocean and the Apex Predators**

Aluminum levels in the ocean vary from 0.01 to 5 ppb. It has been estimated from studies that the major input into the ocean is from aluminum in dust possibly from the atmosphere as we will discuss further on in this chapter. Aluminum input into the ocean is very important because it binds strongly to silicon which then prevents silicon from being absorbed by diatoms. Diatoms are one of the most important algae species in the ocean and they use silicon to form their outer shell. Diatoms are a major base for the food chain in the ocean from which other species depend on for survival. In addition to this, aluminum can actually take the place of silicon in diatoms and pass this aluminum along the food chain to the apex predators such as whales. Right now, whales are dying by beaching themselves at a rate that is 10 times more than what was the case was 20 years ago (https://www.youtube.com/watch?v=L0hsrhNqido). This is definitely related in part to heavy metals such as aluminum and mercury. These days it seems no one has time to talk about such things as vanishing coral reefs and dead whales due to the importance of social media, the threat of war and corona bologna vaccines and their many associated continual, multiple boosters. However, whales are an apex predator and an indicator species, in other words, as they are getting sicker and dying you can bet we are next. I know most people won't understand the importance of that until they are dying as well.

When I had extensively researched mercury toxicity in whales around the world I had determined that the closer marine life is to large cities, the more heavy metals will be found there. This is likely due to the increase in domestic waste as well as the use of heavy metals that are still used in industry and agriculture in most countries.

A study conducted in 2012 had demonstrated that humpback whales off the coast of Maine had elevated levels of aluminum compared to whales found in other parts of the country. The same results were found in the Gulf of Mexico which showed elevated levels of aluminum in three species of whales sampled there which were higher compared to the global average. Stranded killer whales were found in 2015 to contain high levels of aluminum which were associated with higher rates of fungal skin infections and lower levels of selenium and zinc. Selenium and zinc are two necessary minerals that are typically low in mammals that are toxic from heavy metals.

**Freshwater**

Acidic rainfall has contributed to low pH in ponds and lakes causing aluminum to be released from being bound to clay particles in the bottom sediments, resulting in fish kills once the pH drops below 4.5 and the aluminum rises above a level of 1.5 mg/L. When the pH of bound aluminum in the form of chelated hydroxyaluminumsilicate (HAS), or similar compound, drops below 4.7, HAS loses its grip on aluminum and it is released back into the environment. Meanwhile small fish embryos will die when aluminum levels rise above 0.2 mg/L in acidic water. This was a big deal back in the 80s in the US, but not so much now that many coal burning power plants (except Asia of course) were forced to control their noxious sulfur and nitrogen emissions.

**Silica and Oxalate, Two Aluminum Chelators for Plants**

Most agriculture sources will list aluminum toxicity in acid soils as the biggest limitation in expanding soil based agriculture. It has been estimated that 50% of arable land is composed of acidic soils with a pH of less than 5.5 and associated higher levels of aluminum. Aluminum in acid soils causes mineral imbalances and decreases the ability of plants to absorb minerals from the soil (it does the same thing in the human body), while also inhibiting root growth in plants. In addition to what has already been mentioned, excessive acidity in the soil is caused by the use of synthetic sulfur and ammonium-based fertilizers while some soils are naturally acidic and high in sulfur. Maintaining soil pH above 6, through the use of applied lime, while supplementing with silica is an obvious answer to preventing aluminum toxicity in plants as aluminum will chelate with silica and it will remain biologically inactive. Aluminum also binds with oxalic acid (oxalate), which is an organic acid that is toxic when ingested, we will discuss this in greater detail in the next few pages.

Aluminum has no metabolic function in plants and animals and it is toxic to most life on planet earth. It is very important to note here again that separate aluminum ions in any appreciable amount have never been found in an undamaged environment for the past million years on the planet earth as more than 99% of it has been bound to other elements. It is imperative to understand that life on this planet has grown and developed in almost complete absence of appreciable amounts of aluminum ions.

Plants have developed a few ways to deal with the aluminum ions in acid soils. One way is to absorb silica from the soils and make orthosilicic acid (OSA) which is used to bind aluminum into rocks, or phytoliths, within the plants tissue. Because silica binds aluminum so readily and forms a strong bond with it, it can be sequestered into areas of the plant by forming the compound hydroxyaluminumsilicate, rendering it harmless . When we consume these phytoliths in plants, they help us absorb more aluminum that we take in through our diet.

Another way plants adapt to increasing free aluminum ions ($AL^{+3}$) in soils that are acidic is to create compounds called oxalates. Oxalates also bind aluminum so that it cannot create toxicity within the plant and plants increase the amount of oxalates they make in response to increasing aluminum in soils. Plants also release oxalates into the soil to bind aluminum while also releasing already bound aluminum oxalates into the soil. These mechanisms allow plants to survive and grow in heavy metal toxic environments. Plants also use oxalate to bind calcium in soils that contain too much calcium, again, so that the environment becomes fit for plant growth. The stored calcium oxalates also function as a source of calcium that plants can use at a later date. Moreover, plants are able to use calcium oxalate crystals to bind heavy metals in soils so that they can survive in heavy metal contaminated environments.

Oxalates are toxic to most life and they compose about 6% on average of the total dry weight of plants. Plants store oxalate compounds to prevent grazing by animals and to avoid infestation by insects. As little as a 3% oxalate concentration in plants is toxic enough to kill grazing animals and animals avoid plants that have too much of these toxins as they generally taste "terrible".

Reports state that about 30% of all the aluminum in acidic soils will be stored in the leaves and the rest in the roots in soils that have a low pH and contain biologically active aluminum. Oxalates have been shown in published experiments to rapidly increase in response to increased exposure to aluminum in soils. Plants such as Taro increase oxalates in their tissues in response to increasing aluminum in soils so that the plant can bind the aluminum and excrete it into the soil as the plant does not accumulate aluminum, but it will have higher oxalates in aluminum rich environments. Low phosphate soils increase oxalate accumulation in plants as well in order to dissolve aluminum phosphate in soils. This means to the average person that it is best to try and eat vegetables grown on soils that are low in heavy metals, high in minerals like silica and have proper amounts of phosphorous, in other words, composted, organic soils. Areas of high aluminum contamination should be avoided.

Soil fungi use oxalates to chelate heavy metals as well so they are taken out of the soil, "biologically speaking". So, it is obvious that fungi can have a beneficial effect on soils with toxic heavy metals. Fungi work with plants to exchange beneficial compounds which can help remove a certain amount of aluminum in a toxic aluminum environment, but the consequence may be a high oxalate concentration in the edible parts of some plants creating toxicity and inflammation in the human body when consumed.

**Aquatic Animals**

It has been determined through research that aquatic animals will do the same thing as plants to protect themselves from aluminum in the environment. Aquatic animals such as snails will absorb OSA from the water and store it in the form of cellular storage sites called lysosomes. The stored OSA binds to aluminum and it is again stored in a lysosome, preventing the aluminum from becoming toxic, just like what happens in plants.

**Oxalates and Toxicity in Humans**

Unfortunately, oxalate is an anti-nutrient and it can become toxic in the human body when consumed. Some foods that are typically known for their nutritional value and considered "healthy", have high oxalates and should be potentially avoided by anyone detoxing from heavy metals with an already high amount of inflammation in their body.

A person typically ingests about 250 mg of oxalates (oxalic acid) per day and it is rare to have it build up to excessive levels because it is a normal product of metabolism. It can only be removed through urination in functioning kidneys and sweating. Good gut bacteria also break down oxalates while a leaky gut can cause excessive concentrations of oxalates to "leak" into the blood. Candida in the gut can actually create oxalates, however, about 90% of oxalates are absorbed in the stomach.

The primary concern for humans to avoid excessive oxalate intake from plants is to prevent kidney stones from forming due to calcium oxalate precipitation, in those people who are predisposed to developing kidney stones which is about 10% of the population. A diet low in oxalate is one that has less than 50 mg per day. About 80% of all kidney stones formed in the human body are from calcium oxalate formation.

The oxalate content in some plants has become so high that they have become toxic to eat, as aluminum concentrations increase in soil. While most oxalates exist in plants as calcium oxalate, plants also contain soluble oxalates. Fortunately, we don't absorb the calcium oxalate from plants and calcium in our body can bind the soluble oxalates in the gut so it is advisable to eat food that contains calcium when you are eating foods that might contain high amounts of oxalates. The oxalate forms that predominantly exists in the human body are sodium and potassium oxalates.

According to Dr. Sally Norton who is an authority on oxalates in the diet, excessive oxalate intake can cause problems with inflammation, causing extended times to heal from injury, pain, insomnia, brain fog and cognitive disorders and interference with detoxification pathways. All problems already encountered with heavy metal toxicity. The oxalates interfere with cell membranes and energy production in the mitochondria. Further to this, oxalates cause greater histamine release from mast cells increasing pain from inflammation. For someone who has many of these symptoms already, it is obvious there is a great need to avoid some of the high oxalate foods discussed in the next section.

Foods that are typically high in oxalate content are all from plant matter consisting of beets, spinach, some nuts, leeks, okra, sweet potatoes, soy, buckwheat, wheat bran, figs, elderberries, starfruit and rhubarb. The biggest offenders by far seem to be spinach, buckwheat and rhubarb which can typically contain five times more oxalate than rice or millet. Luckily, plant oils and fats are free of oxalates.

Plants make oxalates from vitamin C in response to high levels of metals in the soils or if they have high levels of damage from insects and fungal infections. So, it is obvious that healthy looking plants grown on healthy soils are healthier for you. People that take high amounts of vitamin C may form oxalates from it and this is especially the case if you have high iron and copper in your body and low vitamin B6. Oxalates can also chelate the good metals in your body.

The following list are important points about oxalates that need to be remembered:

1) Oxalates and oxalic acid have been found in air pollution.
2) The thyroid is the main organ where oxalates are stored but sometimes oxalates can be stored in the joints and muscles and cause pain.
3) It is a good idea to avoid some of the high oxalate foods during detox when you already have high amounts of inflammation and engage in an elimination diet to determine if certain foods cause an increase in symptoms.
4) Processing the oxalate depletes the body of B6 so it is a good idea to supplement with this inexpensive vitamin as well as magnesium.
5) Oxalates are primarily removed in sweat and urine.

**Aluminum Toxicity in Bees**

Honey bees are an essential part of the ecology of plants as they help in the reproduction of plants by transferring pollen. Unfortunately, bee numbers have been decreasing for decades and this phenomenon has been labeled colony collapse disorder. According to recently published research, very high levels of aluminum have been found in pollen up to 670 mg/kg. Bees have no taste aversion to aluminum and so they accumulate it in their tissues and it has been reported in scientific publications that during experiments, aluminum in pollen significantly decreases the lifespan of bees compared to control bees that had access to pollen without aluminum.

**In the Air**

For decades I have been listening to first-hand accounts of people talking about chemtrails in various podcasts. Chemtrails are exhaust fumes dispersed from specialized devices on planes that distribute heavy metals into the atmosphere which allow weather manipulation by energizing aluminum particles in the air, from installations such as HARP in Alaska and who knows how else. According to the major source of information on chemtrails, geoengineeringwatch.org, people began seeing chemtrails in the late 1990s.

After studying the 2-hour documentary, "The Dimming", I had to address this heavy metal input that seemed impossible to ignore. The evidence presented by geoengineeringwatch.org is impressive. There are patents you can read about on the internet that relate the distribution of chemicals from airplanes and others that openly discuss equipment for weather manipulation. The evidence that has been documented in this video will likely influence anyone to at least investigate this phenomenon further, regardless if you have never seen a chemtrail or if you think it is a conspiracy theory because you choose to ignore this phenomenon in particular, or if you choose to be ignorant.

This video is hard to find on YouTube and you need a link to view it. The documentary provides many pictures and videos of planes distributing various substances into the atmosphere that can be seen as a "chemtrail". Dane Wigington, who is the lead researcher for geoengineeringwatch.org, begins this documentary by talking about how chemtrails differ from condensation or contrails that are sometimes briefly seen being released out of the regular exhaust of some flying planes. Chemtrails can be seen lingering for hours while contrails disburse readily within minutes. This is widely discussed by flight engineering experts from various sources during the documentary. The "dimming" refers to the light scattering effect, or shading, by these particles, containing aluminum, released as "chemtrails".

Dane Wigington and his team of scientists hired a plane that possessed equipment on board for collecting nano-sized particulates in the atmosphere. Once located, the readily visible chemtrails were observed for hours and the research plane flew through the particulate clouds in the atmosphere and collected atmospheric samples repeatedly during this time.

The collected samples were analyzed for small particulate aluminum and it was confirmed that the chemtrails sampled contained nano-sized particulates composed of aluminum hydroxide. The aluminum particulates can also be found in the blood of people who live on the ground directly below. The blood of the people sampled was determined to be 100 times more than the concentration of any other toxic compound or heavy metal and this level can only be obtained through injection and/or inhalation (Dr. Dietrich Klinghardt, geoengineeringwatch.org). Besides the expected toxicity described here, information from a video on geoengineeringwatch.org also describes how aluminum in the blood finds its way into the mitochondrion, which is the powerhouse of the cell, and creates chronic disease.

Nano-sized aluminum particles do not exist in nature. They have been created artificially. This manmade source of aluminum that is sprayed into our atmosphere has a strong affinity for one of the most widely dispersed toxins in the world, glyphosate. Glyphosate is a manmade chemical that was originally designed to be a heavy metal chelator in the late 1960s, it was not intended to be an herbicide. The other is fluoride which has an amazing history of toxicity that I describe in this book. Aluminum reacts with fluoride to form aluminum fluoride which is another very toxic compound that accumulates in our pineal gland, causing calcification while reducing its ability to function normally.

**Aluminum Absorbed Through the Nose and Lungs**

Aluminum is absorbed through the olfactory route directly into the brain as nasal cavities have a great capacity for absorption. Inhaled aluminum has a direct transit to the hippocampus, which is the area of the brain associated with motivation, emotion, learning, and memory. This toxicity sounds like it could be associated with depression, autism, and Alzheimer's. In human studies, aluminum found in the brains of Alzheimer's patients accumulated in the hippocampus, medial temporal and the frontal cortex, all areas that are associated with memory and facial recognition.

The lungs by their very nature have a large surface area with an incredible capacity for absorption. This renders them overtly acceptable to absorbing aluminum through the air which is eventually transferred by mucus secretions to the gut. An unusual example of this is a research study of people who visited volcanoes taking urine samples before and after. People showed much higher aluminum in their urine after visiting an active volcano compared to urine samples taken before they were exposed to toxic volcanic plumes. In addition, aluminum can enter the lungs from particulates from the burning of fossil fuels. Remember how gasoline for cars used to contain lead? It was taken out because people were getting sick from it.

## Aluminum Production and the Environment

Hmmm.... And once again another unknown source of aluminum in the air we breathe is from the combustion of aircraft and rocket fuel, some of which is dumped just before a plane lands.

In the Mount Shasta region of California, a USDA biologist Francis Mangel had tested the aluminum concentration of water and soil and according to internet sources, determined it contained an average of 4, 610 ppm, which would be 25, 000 times the recommended safe limit (WHO, World Health Organization).

Reports state that there are 42 countries that have engaged in distributing chemicals and metals in the atmosphere.

# Chapter 3

## Sources of Aluminum Toxicity

**Aluminum in Water and Drinks**

In the US, the most widely used water treatment compound to remove particles and make water "cleaner" is aluminum sulfate. This is the main factor contributing to the 0.1 ppm amount of aluminum in over half of the drinking water consumed in that country. Meanwhile OSA levels in the US average only 11 mg/L in drinking water while the average aluminum content is 31 **ppb** in ground water. Aluminum sulfate has been used in water treatment for over 100 years and its use has been steadily increasing ever since.

A sad fact is that many 3rd world people today use aluminum cookware and this is one of the most dangerous sources of aluminum. According to an article in the journal Science of the Total Environment published in 2010, a person who regular uses aluminum cookware can receive 125 mg of aluminum with one serving in each meal. This was actually measured through experimentation. Meanwhile it is important to keep in mind that the WHO recommends an upper limit of 20 mg of aluminum intake per day for a 70 kg adult.

## Aluminum Detox

Fortunately, contact with aluminum foil for untreated and cooked foods does not create any measurable amount of aluminum contamination. Beer in aluminum cans has been measured in scientific studies to contain 0.5 mg of aluminum in each liter of beer consumed while storing the beer at room temperature will significantly increase the aluminum content. Refrigerating canned beer will decrease the amount of aluminum that accumulates in the liquid. Also, brands may differ by a factor of 5 in how much aluminum is transferred from the can to the beer. However, compared to most of the sources of aluminum discussed in this book, canned beer is definitely a minor source. Also, most beers contain orthosilicic acid which strongly binds aluminum and it is removed with urination and sweat.

Tea is very resistant to aluminum and it can absorb a lot of alunimum from the soil, however, this amount can be variable as one scientific report stated that tea leaves can contain up to 30 g of aluminum per kg of dry weight. This is one of the highest concentrations of aluminum in any food item. However, it depends on how much aluminum is found in the soil. In a study conducted in 1997, it was shown through the measurement of aluminum in tea and coffee as well as the transfer of aluminum to the infusion (drink), the amounts were incredibly variable. Coffee was found to be very low in aluminum at 19 ug/g (micrograms per gram) while black tea was very high at 899 ug/g (ppm). It is important to note that when the transfer of aluminum from the tea leaves to the drink was measured, black tea transferred 30% while coffee only had 5% transfer. Even though black tea seems like a poor choice for someone wanting to avoid aluminum in their diet, the consumption of black tea only contributes just 4.2 mg/L of aluminum to a persons aluminum burden according to reports. This amount is likely only less than 10% (1 cup) of the total average daily intake for aluminum in the modern world. The website nutritionfacts.org would concurr with these findings stating that although the consumption of 4 cups of tea can contribute to a full days limit of aluminum, it is likely that only 10% of that is absorbed.

**Aluminum in Food**

The European Food Safety Authority has designated the limit for the allowable weekly aluminum intake in food to be 1 mg/kg of body weight. This is a very high amount. However, humans generally ingest between 1 and 10 milligrams of aluminum everyday through regular whole food consumption and this is not considered to be a potential threat compared to what you might inadvertently consume through aluminum cookware and additives in foods and medicine. Aluminum additives in products such as cheese, salt and grains are major dietary inputs for most people in more modern countries. Eating processed foods regularly can contribute 24 mg of aluminum to the diet per day.

Another source listing the aluminum content of food indicated that adults take in between 9 and 14 mg of aluminum per day from food soruces while for children it is typically half that amount. Infant milk based formulas contain 10 times the aluminum normally found in food while soy based formulas have 25 times the aluminum found in regularly consumed foods. The amount of aluminum that can be absorbed in the intestine from food and liquids can vary by a factor of 10x and some sources state it is about 30% on average. Certain dietary factors such as citrate affect the absorption of aluminum in the diet by binding it.

Aluminum salts are added to many processed foods under the guise that it is harmless. There are many examples of aluminum used as additives in foods. One of the most harmful would be the addition of aluminum in milk and baking powders to prevent clumping. Another example is the addition of aluminum sulfate to white bread as a whitener. An additional and more insane example would be the use of aluminum hydroxide as a baste for large pretzels. The maximum allowable level in foods such as pretzels and baked goods is set at 10 mg/kg (milligrams of aluminum per kilogram of product) according to some well- known, food scientists of Germany. The aluminum in these products can also come from aluminum baking pans dipped in lye. Yuck.

One of the biggest contributors of aluminum to the diet from processed foods is from cheese on frozen pizza which contains up to 14 mg of aluminum per serving. Restaurant pizza normally has cheese of better quality that contains

## Sources of Aluminum Toxicity

10% of that amount. Even that pales in comparison to the insane 72-180 mg of aluminum per serving from ready to eat pancake mixes. However, yet again, although it seems that 30% is absorbed through the gut, it has been reported that the bioavailability is very low (0.1%), but this would typically result in doubling the concentration of aluminum in urine, for a person with good functioning kidneys.

Grains are another food that are typically higher in aluminum content than most, however, the content of aluminum in each type of grain can differ by a factor of 10. Rice and millet were determined to be the lowest in aluminum content at 1.5 to 2.2 mg/kg (milligrams per kilogram, equal to ppm). In contast to this whole wheat and soybeans were 9.6 and 7.1 mg/kg. However, the aveage intake of wheat is about 100 g, so you can figure your daily intake of aluminum from wheat is only about 1 mg or about 10% of the total for a normal, healthy diet. Buckwheat has adapted to high aluminum content in soils and has an aluminum content in leaves as high as 15 g/kg (grams per kilogram) but aluminum is excluded in its seeds through accumulation of oxalate and so the part of the buckwheat plant that is consumed has a concentration of only 3 mg/kg. Corn has an average aluminum content at 4.6 mg/kg.

Certain types of herbs and spices contain more alumnium than others, but the consumption of these inputs is variable as well the aluminum content of each type. According to the avialable scientific literature, spices

**Table 1. Sources of aluminum intake for the human body. The important sources are in bold.**

| Sources of Aluminum | Average Al | Measure |
|---|---|---|
| **Tap water** | **0.1** | **mg/L** |
| Antiperspirants | 70 | mg |
| **Medicine - antacids** | **500** | **mg/tab** |
| Vaccines | 0.125 | mg/shot |
| **Aluminum cookware** | **125** | **mg/serv** |
| Food containers | 16 | mg/L |
| Aluminum cans | 0.5 | mg/L |
| e-cigarettes | 0.05 | mg/day |
| Sunscreen | 200 | mg |
| Turmeric | 0.55 | mg/g |
| Non-dairy creamer | 1.5 | mg/packet |
| **Processed food** | **24** | **mg/day** |
| Tea - Drink | 2 | mg/cup |
| Whole wheat | 1 | mg/100g |

contain a range of aluminum from 50 to 640 ppm or ug/g. The surprise here is that tumeric was reported to have the highest aluminum content at an average of 550 ug/g. This means if you supplement with tumeric as an anti-inflammatory as I do regularly at 1 g per day, which seems to be the suggested dose, than you would be getting about 0.5 mg of aluminum which would be about 5% of the daily intake for someone who does not consume a lot of processsed foods.

## Sources of Aluminum Toxicity

A regular source of aluminum intake that most people would never consider is through crops that are grown on acidic soils. Lower pH in soils facilities an increase in plant uptake of aluminum. Plants such as soybeans tolerate high levels of aluminum in their tissues and these plants can become significant sources with regular ingestion. Soybeans are also high in oxalates. It is important to go organic whenever possible. Organic farmers grow food using healthy soils that have a regular pH and low toxicity.

Another unknown source of toxicity is from the application of aluminum-based herbicides, fungicides and pesticides. A dangerous fact is that the ubiquitous and incredibly toxic herbicide glyphosate found in Round-Up Ready herbicide is a strong aluminum binder. As nearly all Americans have been reported to have glyphosate in their blood due to the incessant and ubiquitous use of this herbicide, it is important to note that when glyphosate binds to aluminum it can cross the blood brain barrier and damage nerve cells. I am going to cover this topic in great detail in my next book.

The original application of glyphosate was for use as a heavy metal binder. An important note here is that glyphosate is a strong chelator of iron, cobalt, copper and molybdenum and these are essential elements for normal functioning human metabolism. Mineral deficiencies have already been widely reported in the last decade to be the root cause of most chronic disease. I wrote about extensively in my book, *Mercury, The Ultimate Truth and Chronic Disease.*

Glyphosate has been associated with damage to the intestinal lining and diseases such as Crohn's disease and irritable bowel syndrome are the rise in most modern countries. These diseases work synergistically with oxalate and aluminum which will become more absorbable with a leaky gut and low levels of beneficial bacteria.

**Aluminum in Antiperspirants**

Research on the absorption rate of aluminum through the skin is scant. However, there is ample evidence supporting the relationship between using underarm antiperspirants and aluminum concentration near the underarm area, and also evidence associating aluminum accumulation in breast tissue and breast cancer. In 2005, a scientific paper published in the Journal of Inorganic Biochemistry stated specifically that underarm antiperspirants have been determined to be linked to the prevalence of breast cancer in numerous studies. The association of breast cancer closest to the underarm area and aluminum accumulation near the underarm area in people using aluminum-based deodorant/antiperspirants as reported by scientific articles, has actually increased over time with the increase in use of aluminum-based deodorants/antiperspirants, increasing from 30% in 1926 to 64% in 1994. The use of aluminum deodorants and antiperspirants increased from $60 billion dollars in sales in 2012 to $80 billion in 2021.

## Sources of Aluminum Toxicity

Aluminum found in antiperspirants is in the form of aluminum chlorohydrate which readily dissolves when applied to underarms and it releases compounds that cause the liberated aluminum to inhibit the release of sweat from sweat glands. Aluminum salts are used in deodorants because they are efficient at reducing sweat production but are aluminum containing antiperspirants really a toxic necessity? In today's insanely busy and stressful world, complete with an adversity to bad smells, deodorants are obviously mandatory, especially in a crowded workplace. However, if anyone took the time to investigate how toxic aluminum in antiperspirants really are, they would never use them again. Fortunately, information regarding aluminum absorption from underarm deodorants is becoming widely available through a series of books released in the last few years that are a mandatory read for anyone wanting to understand why you need to avoid the many toxic effects of this ubiquitous heavy metal.

The amount of aluminum salts from deodorants that actually penetrate the skin is normally very low at 0.01 %, however, the amount of aluminum in these products is high at 5 to 7 percent which results in a relatively high amount of aluminum input into the body. Overall, the amount of aluminum applied to the body in a single application of antiperspirant is in the order of 70 mg.

# Aluminum Detox

## Aluminum in Medicine

The amount of aluminum ingested from pharmaceutical use is considered to be 100 times more than that ingested with food. About one in three people suffer from some sort of heartburn or acid reflux during their lifetime. About 25% of these people suffering from this condition will end up taking an over-the-counter antacid. A very high amount of aluminum is unknowingly ingested with antacids to control chronic disease problems such as acid reflux. Each tablet typically contains 500 mg of aluminum. The crazy part in the use of aluminum antacids is that the manufacturers of this deadly over-the-counter medication actually list in the package that regular consumption of this product should be avoided as it may cause neurological disease like Alzheimer's. Geez how about that? An admission of the connection between aluminum and Alzheimer's. This connection is routinely denied by all researchers working in the field of pharmaceutical drugs. Maybe someone should send them some samples? Something like this would be the response from the medical meatheads "Oh Hey Johnson! Have you've seen what just arrived in the mail today! Free cherry flavored antacid tablets! And woah! Oh BOY! Do they taste yummy! Only 15 calories per tab! No kidding! Crunch. We need to send out a thank you letter! This ought to help my night time reflux problem and hey geez they are free in the mail! My reflux meds are giving me gas and had me shitting the bed the other night! HAHAHHAHA. No kidding…Woah you wouldn't believe the hell my wife gave me"

## Sources of Aluminum Toxicity

There is even a more deadly example of aluminum used in medicine. Aluminum phosphate binders such as aluminum hydroxide are given to patients with poor kidney function as they cannot break down phosphates in the body. The aluminum that travels into the blood crosses the blood-brain barrier causes encephalopathy. On top of this, as lots of water is used to wash away toxins in the blood during dialysis, the semi permeable membrane used in dialysis works both ways with pollutants in the water such as aluminum, entering the blood of dialysis patients through the membrane resulting in dementia like symptoms once crossing the blood brain barrier. Remember that research studies on mammals show that 85% of the aluminum intake that is not excreted ends up in the brain.

Another unknown source of aluminum toxicity is the use of aluminum salts in pharmaceutical drugs. In addition, antibiotics such as Fluoroquinolones bind to aluminum in the gut and increase aluminum uptake in the intestines. This can also occur by changing the natural gut flora leading to increases in fungal populations which create root like structures that invade the intestinal wall causing the well-known leaky gut syndrome. There are numerous scientific reports that show the significant correlation between the overuse of antibiotics and poor mental health.

Other unknown sources of aluminum used in medicine would be aluminum in prosthetics such as hip replacements and dental work. Replacing hips and knees are an everyday thing all over the world, but this is new phenomenon associated with mineral deficiencies and osteoporosis. Increasing aluminum contact in the body only increases mineral deficiencies.

Aluminum in tobacco may not be a significant source of aluminum toxicity due to the fact that people just don't smoke like they used to, after all it is bad for you! However, Dr Chris Exley in his outstanding book *Imagine You Are An Aluminum Atom* had shown through experimental research that absorbing aluminum from heating elements in vaping e-cigarettes results in a higher intake of aluminum in the lungs than smoking Tobacco! That was a shock to me as most people consider vaporing harmless. However, upon closer examination of this, I found research papers stating that it would likely result in less than 1 mg per day with moderate use. However, this form of aluminum may be much more inflammatory.

**Aluminum in Vaccines**

Well hardly anyone in the world today doesn't know about the corona bologna vaccine. Yes that's right citizens step right up and get your third booster to prevent this blatant weak viral disease that seems to be much less damaging than the common flu yet the wonderful governments of the world are chomping at the bit to make it mandatory in order to travel, enter another country and maybe one day enter a supermarket. Major media lies about the number of fatalities from this virus and the so-called vaccine given to people to prevent the disease. The fatalities from the vaccine are another book entirely.

Mercury in vaccines has a 100-year history and mercury is no longer put in vaccines because it was overwhelmingly proven to be the cause of autism. So, the powers that be decided that it was time to bring up another evil: aluminum. Aluminum is added to vaccines as an adjuvant meaning that it elicits an inflammatory immune response. This means that it motivates the immune system to create a war against anything it considers to be a threat. This is currently resulting in an over-inflammatory process contributing to blot clots and autoimmune disorders causing chronic disease and death. I seem to remember that the so-called corona virus did this on its own. The unfortunate part about aluminum in vaccines is that once the body is alerted to the aluminum threat the over-reactive immune cells and associated antibodies continue to identify aluminum as a threat over time and the inflammatory response is elevated and continued. I seem to remember the excitatory phrase "cytokine storm" in relation the media's description of how the corona bologna was causing health problems. So, the solution presented by the darkside is the same one causing problems as the problem itself. Hardly anyone is paying attention to this fact. Create the problem and present the solution, making money going in and make money going out. Geez, these guys don't fool around.

## Aluminum Detox

Once a vaccine containing aluminum is injected into muscle tissue it creates lots of inflammation and this incites specialized white blood cells called macrophages to begin attaching to and transporting the inflammatory aluminum away from the injection site. The aluminum adjuvant is dissolved by the white blood cells and releases super reactive aluminum into the blood or alternatively the cells may even transfer the aluminum cargo directly into the brain resulting in symptoms of autism, Alzheimer's or dementia. This was directly shown by scientific research to be the case in mice injected with aluminum rich vaccines, the marked aluminum was found in the brain. This was then collaborated with studies showing children who died of autism with extraordinarily high levels of aluminum in their brains. Wasn't one of the symptoms of the corona bologna short term memory loss? What a tangled web they have weaved. The rates of autism for a long time have doubled every five years. There are many new names that are now referred to as autism.

Bert Ehgartner in his very detailed book, *The Age of Aluminum*, describes many instances where vaccines were proven to be more effective without the aluminum adjuvant. In the country of Guinea in Africa, children receiving vaccines for measles without any aluminum adjuvant demonstrated increased resistance to other diseases associated with diarrhea, pneumonia and malaria. Most of the book is dedicated to describing how vaccines do not need aluminum as an adjuvant to be successful in preventing disease, in fact, adjuvants were determined to have an ill effect on health.

Studies cited in the *Age of Aluminum* discuss how aluminum containing vaccines administered to people actually resulted in an increased death rate compared to those people not receiving any vaccine. There were repeated negative effects discovered from receiving the diphtheria, tetanus or whooping cough vaccines that contained dead viruses and toxic aluminum adjuvant which could increase your chance of death ten times over. This reminds me of the current situation in regards to the corona bologna, where people receiving the vaccine and booster shots are getting sick with a multitude of strange symptoms similar to the corona virus. HOW STUPID. Here in Panama vaccine givers go house to house with the police and try to tell you it is mandatory, but people who have functioning brains use them to refute the claims and enforce their right of refusal. Some engage in the gross and prolific use of profanities, Oh My!

Vaccines containing live but attenuated viruses (viruses that have been altered so they don't cause disease), activate a different immune system pathway than dead viruses that contain aluminum adjuvant. Live vaccines promote the Th1 pathway which releases the effective cytokines known as interleukin and interferon. Aluminum adjuvants injected into humans invoke the Th2 pathway which causes different results in creating inflammatory conditions from totally different immune cells that are activated.

Once the Th2 pathway is initiated and the over-inflammatory process begins, it can cause pain all over the body in those people who are poor aluminum detoxifiers. This condition is known as macrophagic myositis. Dr. Chris Shade in his videos describes these "poor detoxifiers" as those incapable of excreting heavy metals at a sufficient rate to avoid getting sick from the many heavy metal inputs they receive. The total number was estimated to be about 30% of the total population.

It has been estimated that there are 80 such autoimmune diseases that can form from super reactive immune responses created by injecting aluminum adjuvants. Most of these conditions result from the body's inability to turn off the inflammatory response due to the overinflated reaction from the incredibly toxic and unnecessary aluminum. The antibodies that are formed from the hyper inflated inflammatory signals sometimes attach to the body's own tissues causing serious tissue damage. These conditions continue until the aluminum is completely removed from the body. The good news is that it is much easier to do than mercury. I will describe all of the many facets of aluminum detox in chapter 8, but first I will continue to finish our story how aluminum causes disease in the human body.

# Chapter 4

## Aluminum and Disease

### Aluminum, The Universal Metabolic Disruptor

Because of the ability of aluminum ions to bind to so many valuable compounds imperative to human biochemistry, it has been branded a "universal metabolic disrupter". The importance of this can be truly understood when one considers that aluminum readily and avidly binds to the most common and most important biologically active molecules in the human body. Oxygen containing molecules, such as the main energy molecule of the human body known as ATP or adenosine triphosphate, can be bound by aluminum. Once bound, the molecule becomes inactive and would obviously contribute to chronic fatigue. The ATP molecule has a strong preference for aluminum and it will bind to this much more readily than its intended metal necessary for it to function, magnesium. The same is true of other heavy metals such as mercury.

Another important molecule for a proper functioning metabolism is carboxylic acid. Carboxylic acid is an important component of proteins and proteins are made up of amino acids, which also contain carboxyl groups. It is easy to see how aluminum can interfere with the human body as it forms strongly bonded compounds with proteins, which are the body's main unit for structure and function.

Aluminum binds to citric acid which is a valuable nutritional acid which helps to prevent kidney stones and is another unreplaceable compound involved in energy production, transferring food energy into cellular energy. In addition, citric acid enhances the bioavailability of minerals, allowing your body to better absorb them in the gut. As heavy metals readily take the place of necessary elements in your body such as magnesium, it seems that aluminum ions attached to compounds such as citric acid have a triple negative effect.

Iron is another important metal for human health that is disrupted by aluminum in at least two different ways. Because aluminum has the same charge and shape as iron it can be transferred past the blood brain barrier attached to a normal glycoprotein carrier found in the blood known as transferrin. This is one way aluminum can quickly get access to the brain. According to a professor of neuro degenerative disease in Australia, Judie Walton, aluminum collects in cells that are iron dependent, dysregulating iron homeostasis and causing microtubule depletion.

**Alzheimer's and Other Neuro Degenerative Disease**

Right now, over 35 million people worldwide suffer from Alzheimer's disease. One in three people over 80 have the disease and will likely die from it within a few years.

# Aluminum and Disease

Standard medical science claims there is no cause and it may be linked to a genetic variation of an APOE gene. This gene is involved in fat binding proteins and its primary function is to deliver cholesterol to the nerve tissue in the brain while also being linked to inflammatory modulation and the associated immune cells. According to the latest peer reviewed scientific studies, those that have this variation have more beta amyloid molecules that attract and attach to aluminum which increases the toxicity of the combination by at least 10 times, thus increasing the likelihood and development of the disease. Moreover, calcium signaling, and proper mitochondrial respiration is strongly disrupted by when aluminum binds to the beta amyloid molecules and this is the trigger identified that causes death of the nerve cells.

Alzheimer's disease was first discovered in 1906. Research looking into the connection between Alzheimer's and aluminum began in 1965 somewhat accidently as scientists were looking to determine something unrelated to Alzheimer's disease. Aluminum adjuvant (aluminum phosphate) was injected into the brains of rabbits to experiment with antibodies and to the surprise of the scientists conducting the experiment, neuro degenerative microfibrillary tangles, classically associated with Alzheimer's disease, developed. Since then, further investigation has showed this strong association time and again. The only thing stopping an overwhelming amount of investigation into aluminum causing Alzheimer's disease is the lack of grants to support this research as aluminum toxicity is bad for the aluminum and pharmaceutical businesses. Once again, the irony here is that leaders of the aluminum industry serve on the board of directors for Alzheimer's research committees. The word is, is that everyone on that committee gets along swimmingly well. The increase in Aluminum production is incredibly correlated with the increase in the incidence of Alzheimer's from the year 1960 onwards, the figures and data exactly match up.

Analysis of human biopsy tissue shows very strong correlations between the accumulation of aluminum and the increase in age of human beings. This is important when we consider the discussion presented here in regards to what cells actually accumulate aluminum over time. Long lived brain cells such as neurons are main targets for aluminum binding, causing massive amounts of inflammation and eventual destruction.

The myelin sheath surrounding nerve tissue is the inflammatory target of aluminum and thus multiple sclerosis and similar neuro inflammatory diseases have been associated with aluminum concentrations in the brain. Oligodendrocytes which are the cells responsible for the repair of the myelin sheath of nerve cells are one the cells most affected by aluminum toxicity. Once aluminum attaches to the myelin sheath it signals the immune system to begin to attack it, leading to the many different neuro inflammatory diseases such as multiple sclerosis.

## Aluminum and Disease

A series of large epidemiology studies have shown that increased concentrations of aluminum in drinking water had a direct relationship with increasing the likelihood of developing Alzheimer's disease. The same studies also demonstrated that drinking water that contained at least 18 mg/L of orthosilicic acid (OSA) would result in people not developing Alzheimer's disease while contributing to cognitive performance. This relationship will be discussed in the next two chapters.

A study in France conduced over a period of 15 years examined the association of aluminum intake in drinking water and the development of dementia. People who ingested greater than 0.1 mg of aluminum in drinking water had a significantly greater chance of developing dementia compared to those individuals who did not have any alumiunum in the water they drank. Conversely, people who drank water that had greater than 10 mg of silica in the form of orthosilicic acid (OSA) in their drinking water had a decrease in the risk of developing any cognitive decline.

As will be discussed in great length in chapter 9, OSA is the key that will completely reverse the symptoms of Alzheimer's. In another scientific study French researchers concluded that water that was contaminated with aluminum above a level of 0.1 mg/l, from the use of aluminum sulfate in water treatment processes, had doubled the chance of experiencing Alzheimer's disease in those unfortunate individuals drinking it. The data was compared to people drinking tap water that contained little or no aluminum. The EU limit on aluminum in drinking water is double the amount used in this study at 0.2 mg/L.

Daniel Perl, professor of neuropathology in the US, developed an imaging technique that showed the highest concentration of aluminum was found in the middle of the Alzheimer's amyloid beta plaques, which is always considered the hallmark sign of the disease once brain tissues are examined. Aluminum in the brains of Alzheimer's patients accumulates in the hippocampus, medial temporal and the frontal cortex regions, all areas that are associated with memory and facial recognition. The areas most damaged in the brain of Alzheimer's patients contained two to three times more aluminum when compared to people not suffering from the disease. These amyloid plaques cause disruptions in neural transmission and eventually destroy neural tissue. Aluminum interferes with the body's ability to prevent and decrease the formation of amyloid beta plaques, which are an indicator of Alzheimer's disease. Tau proteins normally found inside nerve cells that aid in transport pathways also become tangled and lead to increased toxicity and eventual death of nerve cells in chronically ill Alzheimer's patients.

Not only is aluminum toxic to nerve cells directly, it can also indirectly cause damage. In other brain studies, low concentrations of aluminum can induce the gene expression of pro-inflammatory signals. These inflammatory signals lead to damage in neural tissue resulting in diseases such as Alzheimer's.

The situation is much different for other toxic metals. For example, once your body detects cadmium, special proteins are made to bind and remove cadmium from the body. About 80% of the mercury that you ingest will end up in the kidney, yet enough of this toxic heavy metal gets into the brain, to cause a variety of neuro degenerative diseases. I will eventually report on the toxicity of other heavy metals in more books I will write as time permits.

**Cardiovascular Disease**

Aluminum inhibits the use of stored fat and glucose for energy, increasing the likelihood of developing cardiovascular disease. In addition, a high animal protein diet decreases silica intake which also increases cardiovascular disease. Consuming more vegetables increases OSA content in the body and lowers aluminum. In contrast, aluminum lowers carnitine in the blood. Carnitine increases energy by directing fatty acids to the mitochondrion for oxidation and energy production. The main source of carnitine in the body is from the consumption of red meat. Cardiovascular disease is the number one killer in the US while people dying from stroke is number 5. Remember here we are omnivores, originally hunter/gatherers and we were designed to eat a lot of different types of food.

## Cell Longevity, Osteoporosis and Hip Fractures

Dr Chris Exley is a UK college professor and he is the premier scientist working in the field of aluminum toxicity. His book, *Imagine You Are an Aluminum Atom*, provided much of the cutting-edge information needed to fit the pieces of this puzzle together. This part of the story starts with cells. As previously mentioned, short lived cells in the human body are damaged by aluminum, but they are regularly replaced as part of normal growth and metabolism before they can experience the neuro toxic effects from aluminum. However, longer lived cells like nerve and bone cells are damaged in a more permanent way. When bones tissue is formed, biological fluids containing calcium are made available to increase bone mass. Unfortunately, aluminum readily takes the place of calcium in bones that are forming and the aluminum becomes trapped inside bone tissue. The aluminum ion does the same thing to magnesium with aluminum replacing this valuable element in 100s of normal metabolic reactions in the human body. The same thing happens with mercury.

People knowledgeable about detox are very familiar with the major area of deposition of heavy metals such as lead, which also finds its way into bones and remains there unless removed through processes such as heavy metal detox, which is described in this book and the one I wrote before this one. The irony here is that individuals that are heavy metal toxic are typically mineral deficient as heavy metals prevent the absorption, utilization and transfer of the good metals in the human body such as calcium, magnesium and zinc. This work has been very well described by Dr Andrew Cutler in regards to mercury, in his seminal book *Amalgam Illness, Diagnosis and Treatment*. As the body becomes depleted of essential elements such as calcium, it is removed from the bones as needed rendering them more brittle. This is widely evident in today's elderly where hip, and knee replacements are now the norm and by and large, no longer a rare occurrence.

Another such unfortunate occurrence is the fact that the kidneys are another area of aluminum deposition and cause damage. Once again, the irony here is that heavy metal removal is accomplished by kidneys, the very organ damaged by heavy metals in the first place.

# Chapter 5

## Measuring Aluminum in the Human Body

My experience in measuring heavy metals in the human body has demonstrated time and again that hair samples are invaluable for determining not only what heavy metals are present in the human body but also what minerals are deficient as a result of heavy metal toxicity. By determining mineral deficiencies and overabundance of minerals in the human body, we can see the evidence for the heavy metal toxicity which directly interferes with the regulation of minerals in the blood. We can then supplement accordingly.

It is obvious but worth stating that the use of aluminum rich antiperspirants prevents the use of underarm hair for heavy metal analysis. Better sources are untreated hair from the scalp, face, pubic or hair shaved from legs etc.

Blood represents the vehicle for heavy metal removal as the body quickly removes heavy metals in the blood through regular excretion through the liver and kidneys or by depositing in various tissues such found in the brain, liver and kidney thus complicating and extending detox. When removing heavy metals from the blood through regular detox and chelation, the body's regular functions then release heavy metals from tissues which travel around through the blood for removal. If this process is engaged too intensively, you can inadvertently poison yourself and experience adverse symptoms such as short term memory loss (brain fog), muscle pain, insomnia, chronic fatigue, digestive disorders etc. The best response to this is to engage in liver and kidney detox before continuing with heavy metal removal.

Once you engage in proper detoxification and heavy metal removal through sweat therapy, intestinal binders and liposomal vitamin C, hair testing will readily show the increase in heavy metals representing the increase in the blood over time. Hair analysis typically shows the heavy metal accumulation in the blood from the environment of from your tissues, over a period of about three weeks. Thus, blood is the vehicle in and the vehicle out of the body, but the concentration of heavy metals in the blood varies greatly over time (days) in response to how much is consumed and how much is excreted. So, blood and urine analysis are only a snapshot of the concentration of heavy metals and this amount does not reflect the amount stored in the tissues. A better use of blood and urine analysis is a comparison to see how much is excreted through the urine verses how much is in the blood. For example, if the amount of aluminum in the blood is high and the amount that should be excreted in the kidneys is low, there may be a problem with kidney function.

# Chapter 6

## Aluminum Detox, It's in The Water

People who are full of toxic metals are typically advised to engage in the classically reported to be successful detox protocols, such as sweat therapy and intestinal binders such as chlorella and spirulina oral supplements. My experience over the past decade has also revealed that liposomal vitamin C is imperative both for its effectiveness in reducing oxidative stress caused by mercury and its low cost. Vitamin C increases the concentration of the body's master antioxidant and chelator: glutathione. According to Dr. Chris Shade who could likely be labeled "Mr. Mercury", the increase in the intake of antioxidants in the human body increases the production of glutathione, which together with essential enzymes and carrier proteins gained through proper nutrition, remove bound heavy metals through the gastrointestinal tract (GIT). This is where 80% of all mercury is normally removed, bound to glutathione, and directed through the liver, a main area of glutathione production, through the gall bladder and out with regular, daily waste removal in the GIT. Antioxidants upregulate the genes responsible for glutathione production. Liposomal vitamin C has been reported to be a viable way to increase glutathione production in the human body and it has become a regular component of my detox protocol which has helped my clients remove

# Aluminum Detox

heavy metals and recover from heavy metal toxicity and chronic illness expressed as neural toxicity and immune suppression. If you experience a problem with detoxification according to established protocols it may be better to detox your liver and kidneys first before engaging in serious heavy metal detox.

The good news is that aluminum is by far much easier to remove from the human body compared to mercury which typically takes years and special protocols for those unlucky enough to be seriously mercury toxic. Detoxing aluminum is simple, drink silica in the form orthosilicic acid (OSA) also referred to as silicon. This is widely available in certain mineral waters such as "Fiji" water which contains some of the highest silica rich sources available. It reminds me of the saying "Let Food by Thy Medicine", made famous by Hippocrates, the father of modern medicine. Just as applicable would be "Let water be thy medicine", as this has been documented to be the way to go for those experiencing aluminum toxicity.

When drinking OSA water like that found in "Fiji" and "Vulvic", it is important to drink a certain amount over time. For instance, one glass per day will have a negligible effect but 1.5 liters drunk in one hour will raise the OSA in the blood to bind a significant amount of aluminum that can be readily measured in the urine if a person is sufficiently hydrated and urinates. Within a few hours after drinking OSA water, the amount of aluminum in the blood and in the urine increases to a peak and then declines. It has been proven and documented that drinking OSA water at a rate of 1.5 liters, preferable one cup every three hours, for three months continuously, will significantly reduce stored aluminum in the body.

Well, it seems kind of funny, but, the best sources of silica for the human body are mineral waters and beer. Beer also made an appearance in the book I wrote on mercury toxicity, because it helps to release mercury through the breath for seriously toxic, mercury sufferers like mercury miners. This was amply described in my book on mercury toxicity. Since I like ice cold beer and it seems to be a weakness of mine, I had to laugh at finding this out. But back to our story you can't just get plastered every day to get rid of your aluminum, haahha.

Studies conducted on rats would prove that OSA given at the same time as aluminum in experimental diets would prevent the aluminum from getting attached to nerve cells in the brain, preventing damage. Rats fed diets containing aluminum without any OSA, wound up having aluminum accumulate in the olfactory bulb part of the brain. Upon further analysis it was determined that the OSA not only bound aluminum ions when aluminum and OSA were given together, but the OSA could also remove previously consumed aluminum that was almost all bound in the areas of the brain known as the olfactory bulb and cerebellum. The cerebellum is the area of the brain that controls coordination and movement and when this area is toxified from aluminum, Parkinson's disease develops.

## Aluminum Detox

Minor amounts of aluminum were also found in the bones, spleen, kidney and liver, but it is important to note that these amounts were only 15% percent of the total, meaning 85% of the ingested aluminum ended up in the brain. This is an incredibly important study that shows that OSA is the answer for the PREVENTION AND CURE of neurological disease due to aluminum toxicity. It was shown in a similar study that OSA could actually be directed to the kidneys to prevent aluminum damage there as well.

Silica is necessary for the metabolism of connective tissues. Unlike aluminum, silica is a necessary nutrient for tissue formation and flexibility, in all animals. As animals age, silica is lost from arterial tissues, resulting in arteriosclerosis, while the loss of silica from skin tissue causes wrinkles.

Silica ingested by itself does not pass readily into the blood from the intestine so silica supplements are not expected to help with Alzheimer's. As exotic bottled water drunk daily for months can be expensive it is important to note that it is possible to make a synthetic water containing OSA. Synthetic OSA waters can be created by using a water with a pH of 4.7 and then adding sodium silicate (see books and videos by Dr. Dennis Crouse). However, it is also important to note that only a maximum concentration of 200 mg/L of OSA can be achieved as beyond this the compound will precipitate as colloids and be less available to the human body for binding aluminum for removal. And if not enough water is present to flush the excess OSA out of the body in the event of too much addition of silicates, kidney stones can form, so it is obvious that close attention needs to be paid when making synthetic OSA water. It seems the best way to get rid of aluminum from the body once it has been chelated by silica is through the sweat and urination. Secondly through the GIT.

Sufferers of mercury toxicity who have used the Andrew Cutler protocol are disturbingly familiar with the term half-life when talking about chelators. Chelators are chemical substances that attach to heavy metals in the body for removal. Orthosilicic acid is a chelator. When you drink or eat OSA it passes through the intestine and into the blood and attaches to aluminum. This chelated aluminum is known as hydroxyaluminumsilicate. The half-life of OSA in water is 3 hours. This means that once OSA water is ingested it will bind aluminum for three hours and then it is estimated that 50% of the aluminum will be released back into the blood as free ionic aluminum. For those that are heavy metal toxic, this means redistribution of heavy metals and the potential creation of detox symptoms of aches and pains, fatigue, short term memory loss and other problems which of course adds difficulty to detoxification. If you can't remember to take your chelators how can you detox? Write it down and have alarms.

Dr. Chris Exley demonstrated through clinical trials that the regular intake of OSA water reduced the body burden of aluminum and increased measurable cognitive function in those people suffering from Alzheimer's and dementia. An important note here is that mineral rich waters that contain OSA are in the form of silicon which can pass easily into the blood from the gut and bind aluminum for removal, but the labels on the bottles of water always list silica or orthosilicic acid.

Men excrete more aluminum in their sweat overall because they sweat more than women. Meanwhile both men and women will double the amount of aluminum in their sweat after drinking sufficient amounts of OSA water. Volumes of sweat can exceed 4 liters per hour during heavy exercise and this can equal more than the total amount removed during urination. Women excrete more aluminum in their urine compared to men, so this obviously helps to balance out aluminum removal between the sexes.

Pregnant mothers have been reported to have low levels of OSA in their blood while the concentration of OSA in their growing baby is much higher, indicating a sacrificial relationship which is also seen in pregnant female animals. Moreover, breast milk during the first month of life of the newborn child contains OSA as well. So, it seems that nature finds a way of dealing with the toxicity of aluminum in order to survive.

Once OSA rich water is collected from springs and transferred to reservoirs or ponds the OSA concentration decreases as it attaches to organic matter or algae and settles out in bottom sediments. This is one reason why water is bottled and delivered from the source.

**The Blue Zones, More Irrefutable Proof**

I have previously read the book about the Blue Zones by Dan Buettner. Much of the book relates how people living in certain areas of the planet live longer than average, in particular, where an above average of people live to be more than 100 years old. The book relates the longevity to a variety of factors such as eating more of a plant-based diet, having a "purpose" in life, developing better family relationships etc., and at a minor level, calcium and magnesium in the water they drink. A particular interesting fact is that in the blue zone that is composed of an island off of the coast of Greece, there is almost no dementia. In fact, blue zoners on the whole have a much lower rate of Alzheimer's.

Further to this, the more recently released book that examines the incredible connection between silica rich water and the reduction in chronic disease is *Silica Water, The Secret of Healthy Blue Zone Longevity In The Aluminum Age*. Dr Dennis Krouse, author of the book on silica water in the blue zone, recommends having one glass of OSA water every three hours during the day, which would likely be good for a lot of things as water consumption is an essential method of detox. By keeping aluminum in the blood chemically bound for an extended period of time, the bound aluminum will leave through the kidneys during normal urination. The recommendation for this was from examination of the link between low rates of chronic disease and the natural OSA concentration in the water where people live a very long life on average.

Dr. Dennis Crouse discovered something very unique during his research of blue zones. He discovered that that there was a strong correlation between the longevity of the blue zone people and the OSA concentration in the water they drank. Compared to similar areas that were out of the blue zone, there was only about 25% chance of living past 100. It was revealed that the higher the levels of OSA (silicon) in the drinking water, the more you have the blue zone effect, resulting in a longer life. Blue Zone males living in Sardinia have twice the longevity as mainland Italians.

Lowering the level of aluminum in the blood due to daily drinking of OSA water in the blue zones has shown to result in decreased levels of the inflammatory marker, homocysteine, which then contributes to a decrease of 80% in arteriosclerosis compared to people who are not living in a blue zone. Aluminum interferes with an enzyme that converts homocysteine into the beneficial amino acid methionine.

If you live in the US, there is a five times higher chance of being affected by heart disease and a 7 times higher chance of developing prostate cancer compared to people lucky enough to live in a blue zone. People living on the island of Ikaria have 50% the rate of heart disease compared to Americans.

Aluminum has also been found to interfere with the body's ability to repair DNA and this has been shown to result in blue zones having a breast and prostate cancer rate of 80% less compared to the people living in the US.

Drinking OSA rich water results in a decrease in the loss of minerals in bones as well as an increase in the rate of bone regeneration. This would contribute to people living in the blue zone having less hip fractures, something that occurs at an epidemic rate in the elderly of the US. All of the blue zones are located in areas that get above average amount of sun, so their natural production of vitamin D is likely higher.

When examining the levels of elements in the soil and water in a blue zone of Asia, it was determined that only an increased OSA concentration was related to an increase in longevity while none of the other 12 elements examined seem to play a part in increasing the longevity of the people who live there.

Ok, so to review, various mineral waters contain silica in a form known as orthosilicic acid (OSA) which strongly bonds to or chelates aluminum as the compound known as hyrdroxyaluminumsilicate, which can then excreted by urine, feces or sweat. Studies show fast and incredibly effective aluminum removal for people suffering from symptoms of Alzheimer's. It has been demonstrated that drinking 1.5 liters of mineral water containing at least 30 mg of silica (14 mg of OSA, "Fiji" or "Volvic") per day in the order of about 6 weeks continuously, can reduce the symptoms of Alzheimer's which are always associated with high levels of aluminum in the brain. It is important to bring a magnifying glass with you to check the silica levels in different waters when you buy them at the store because they vary in silica concentration by more than a factor of 10. The amount of OSA in water should be sufficiently high so that aluminum is continually bound until it is removed by the kidneys during regular urination. This amount according to Mr. Aluminum (Dr Chris Exley) is 30 mg/L as silica or half that as OSA.

# Chapter 7

## OSA in the Diet and Other Detox Methods

So how do mammals normally get rid of aluminum without the ingestion of orthosilicic acid (OSA) rich water? A cursory search on the internet for aluminum detox will inform you to simply eat more green beans and that's it. Well, I was skeptical that it could be that easy and this sounded ridiculous, but maybe not. Green beans according to published, peer-reviewed science papers contain a high level of OSA (reported as silica) at 5.5 mg per 100g and with a high absorption rate as well (50%). So, eating more green beans is a good idea for aluminum detox. Also, whole rice and legumes seem to be a good choice. I do not advocate eating processed foods and high carbohydrate foods generally, but I have made the information available in Table 2(next page).

It is imperative to understand that the content of silica (OSA) in food is only half of the information you need to know in order to get the necessary amount of silica from food for the chelation of aluminum, the other half is how much silica is actually absorbed from the food so it can be utilized by the body. An important example of this would be some these straightforward facts: meat has very little silica while mussels and some seafood items are high in silica but have poor absorption. So certain grains and vegetables are your best sources.

It is obvious from what has been reported here that aluminum is toxic to all life and all life should avoid it. Plants absorb silica from the soil when it is available. They use the silica in the soil to form orthosilicic acid in order to bind aluminum to prevent it from being toxic. The bound aluminum is in the form of nano-sized particles known as phytoliths. When we eat plants that are high in silica as phytoliths, it helps to bind aluminum and it leaves through the GIT. The OSA reduces aluminum in the body overall while phytoliths remove aluminum in the gut at a better rate than OSA. So, it seems once again that the consumption of whole vegetables cannot be beat when it comes to increasing health and avoiding chronic disease.

Most of the silica in the edible parts of plants is stored in the skin and hulls and so if you consume the hulls of oats for example you can easily get 10 times more silica than if you just consume the inside, less fibrous parts of the edible plants. Meanwhile processed foods contain very little silica and so this is another reason people who eat processed foods are unhealthy.

Silica is a necessary nutrient that generally decreases with increasing age. Silica is necessary for strong bones and increases the collagen content in bone. Silica deficiency is characterized by brittle nails and hair, poor skin condition and poor calcium absorption. The recommended amounts required in the diet are from 200 to 500 mg per day.

Table 2. Sources of silica in the diet, important sources are in bold.

| Type | mg per 100 g | % absorption |
|---|---|---|
| **Green Beans** | **2.5** | **50** |
| Bananas | 6.1 | 5.8 |
| Spinach | 1.7 | 26 |
| Rice | 8 | 53 |
| Grains | 7.8 | 44 |
| Lentils | 11 | 26 |
| pasta | 1.1 | 58 |
| Fruit | 1.34 | 13 |
| Beans | 5.5 | 0.6 |
| Mussels | 9.6 | 5.5 |
| **Whole oats** | **278** | **49** |
| **Barely** | **109** | **49** |
| **Potatoes** | **93** | **21** |
| Corn | 2 | 49 |

Although the majority of new information strictly focuses on OSA, Klauss Kaufmann in his book titled *Silica The Amazing Gel* focused on studies that showed that people taking sodium silicate along with aluminum in an experimental setting would show no measurable aluminum in the blood while people given dissolved aluminum without any sodium silicate would have measurable amounts of aluminum.

In another study, Belgian researchers determined that Alzheimer's was accelerated by the blockage of arteries in the brain that supplied neural tissue with blood that provided oxygen and nutrition and removed waste. As mentioned before, silica in the body maintains the elasticity of arteries. As silica in its mineral form is largely undigestible, it has been suggested that organic silica from the herb horsetail or a gelatinous silica made from minerals would be more absorbable. Silicic acid is actually hydrated silica, or silica gel.

The most important food crops in the world absorb silica to form OSA in order to bind toxic aluminum. Important widely consumed plants like corn, barley and soybeans accumulate so much silica, that silica can actually total 1% of the total dried weight of the plant. The bound silica aluminum complex is stored in the plant as a hydroxyaluminumsilicate phytolith, until the protection is passed on to the human gut when consumed, or degrades with a low pH environment.

Agricultural sources state that about 50% of vegetable production comes from tropical and subtropical areas that largely have soils of a low pH of about 5.5. The soils from these areas are characteristically low in nutrient content and are greatly affected by heavy metal toxicity such as manganese, aluminum and iron. Aluminum toxicity in soil is considered to be the biggest factor that negatively affects agriculture production. In soils with a neutral pH and minor acidity, aluminum exists as non-reactive and benign forms such as aluminum silicates and aluminum oxides. In contrast to this, soils with low pH, below 6.5, have forms of aluminum that are more toxic. However, the aluminum in these plants is mostly bound with silica.

Irrigation of plants with 50 to 100 mg/l (ppm) silica rich water results in an increase in silica content of leafy vegetables by a factor of 2 to 6 times, but foliar applications are more efficient in the transfer to silica to plants, in other words plants absorb silica through the leaves better than through the roots. Silica fertilizers like magnesium silicate can increase crop yields (sugarcane and others) by 15% and sugar production by 20%.

The human body contains 20 mg of silicon per kg of body weight. The major areas of deposition are bone, tendons, aorta, liver and kidney. Silica is widely known for being important for maintaining healthy connective tissue such as skin and bone. Research published in the British Journal of Nutrition clearly states that silica intake through the diet is strongly correlated with bone density. This is easily understood as there are at least 10 different minerals involved in bone formation, so taking calcium when you are mineral deficient is not a good idea as excess calcium in the blood along with arterial inflammation is associated with forming arterial plaques and arteriolosclerosis. So, it is best to take a full range mineral supplement if you find you have deficiencies through a hair test analysis.

## Aluminum Detox

Published peer-reviewed studies state that people that have been diagnosed with MS are known to excrete high levels of aluminum through their urine while having a documented higher than average total body burden of aluminum accumulation. Surprisingly, EDTA which is a chelator that was originally associated with lead removal, has been shown to increase aluminum in the urine after IV treatment along with an increase in antioxidants. Antioxidants are known to increase glutathione production, the body's own master chelator.

In a detox book called *Dirty Genes*, Dr Ben Lynch stated that the genes responsible for detoxification can be upregulated or "turned on" by eating a better diet including leafy greens which also donate methyl groups bound to the vitamin folate which then drives proper metabolism and detoxification. Dr Chris Shade in his video lectures would concur with these findings as he stated the increased consumption of antioxidants would cause an upregulation of an NRF2 protein which genetically "turns on" the production of glutathione and increases the body's ability to remove mercury, predominantly through the GIT. So, it seems vegetables are the best thing for you. Silica removal from the blood is accomplished by the kidney and urine can give an indication of silica absorption through the diet.

## Ionic Foot Baths

When researching ionic foot baths for the potential to remove heavy metals in the human body, I did not find much information during the year of 2018 when I did most of my writing for my mercury book. The few studies I did find were either inconclusive or the results indicated that the saltwater baths that had a minor amount of DC current running through them did not collect any heavy metals from the human body. The truth is that the steal electrodes used in the ionic foot baths oxidize and it turns the water brown, in other words, rust. Many so-called health practitioners will tell you that the water is full of toxins from your body (this is what happened to me in Boquete, Panama). This is not true at all. Scientific studies that have actually measured the water for heavy metals with and without any human contact have shown that the metals in the water come from the machine and not the human body. However, after watching a video from geoengineeringwatch.org, I was convinced to have another looks at ionic foot baths in their ability to help the human body detox from heavy metals.

According to Dr. Dietrich Klinghardt, the use of the ionic footbath activates the kidneys, which are then able to eliminate heavy metals through urination. So this may be from the electrical current in the body stimulating the removal of heavy metals from tissues and then the body's own glutathione binding the aluminum for removal while the electrical current may provide electrons for an antioxidant effect as well. In other words, it works like an "extractor", freeing metals up to be removed through circulation in the blood and aiding the removal. I had experienced a similar effect when eating raw coriander in 2018. Unfortunately, at that time I had so much mercury in my body as this was the beginning of detox that it gave me horrible brain fog and fatigue.

There is an associated between Wi-Fi and aluminum toxicity. Wi-Fi and excess electromagnetic radiation reduce electrons in the human body. We are continually surround by it and it is set to get more intense with the advent of 5G and the increased amount of energy necessary to get the smaller wavelength signals to travel farther. Once the body is in a state of reduced electrons, aluminum becomes even more toxic. One way to increase electrons is through the already mentioned above, ionic foot baths, and another way is earthing, in other words connecting your body to the ground, either directly or by attaching a conductive pad to your body which is attached to a wire that is inserted in the ground. This is done to allow the body to absorb electrons from the earth which is negatively charged and full of electrons.

**Glutathione, The Chelator the Body Makes**

I did find a few studies demonstrating that glutathione removes aluminum in the same way it removes other heavy metals. Studies published in peer-reviewed journals show that glutathione is activated in accordance with increased aluminum levels. Other studies show repeatedly that glutathione is reduced with the increased ingestion of aluminum. To verify the idea that glutathione is binding aluminum for removal, aluminum would have to be measured in the urine or through the GIT and these studies may yet to have been undertaken. But what about the everyday aluminum removal strategy? Well, it goes back to diet, let food and water be thy medicine.

Glutathione is found in nearly all foods. Published research has determined that food derived glutathione can be found in the blood and liver of those that consume it. Daily consumed glutathione through the ingestion of whole foods averages about 35 mg per person per day. A study published in the journal of Nutrition and Cancer in 1994 revealed that glutathione content of food was highest for vegetables, and vegetables are the highest source of antioxidants and so this is another reason to eat more vegetables! In addition to this, another study from 2015 published in the European Journal of Nutrition demonstrated that oral supplementation of glutathione increased the body's reserves of glutathione, decreased oxidative stress and doubled the effectiveness of the body's natural killer cells. Glutathione also chelates heavy metals and so it seems to be a big part of the solution for survival on this planet for the human species.

# Chapter 8

## Conclusion, Depopulation and the End Game

China, of course, has increased its aluminum production by a factor of 10 times during the last decade. This is only adding to the environmental disaster that has become that country's identity. Worldwide aluminum production is scheduled to double in the next 20 years, and it will likely find its way into more products at a higher concentration.

The cause of neuro degenerative disease is known and it can be prevented and cured. It is hard to believe that knowledge could prevent the scheduled increase in Alzheimer's and save 100s of millions of lives. What would anyone have to lose by trying the detox methods mentioned in this book and others, and engaging in recovery? Not much. However, people have everything to lose in terms of their financial stability, emotional stress, destruction of family and of course the loss of life.

So, when you are a hardcore researcher like me and you get to the point where you think you know most everything that is going on about a particular subject, in other words you have come out of the rabbit hole, you find yourself wondering not so much how did it all happen and where is it all going but rather why? Why is there so little concern about human health and welfare and so much focus on accumulating wealth? A certain number of people can detox adequately enough to remove a sufficient amount of aluminum and other heavy metals so that they don't really get sick until a threshold is reached and then there is a big crash. I am familiar with this when I work with Rife technology to cure people from chronic disease as 80% of the people I see have real problems with their health and they are searching for the cheap, magic bullet that will get them back into their old life of doing whatever they want. Most people don't want to learn about this stuff until they have to.

So, what is the end game? Easy. Just read information about the Georgia guide stones, Agenda 21/30, new world order etc. The end game is depopulation. It is about control, power and influence. This is why the medical industry focuses on keeping most everyone sick, on drugs and uniformed. Let us go back to the data and bring this idea home to give some final thoughts and develop an idea of where we need to go from here.

Unfortunately, semen accumulates aluminum more so than what can be found in the blood and this results in a reduction in sperm count for those unfortunate males stricken with aluminum toxicity. The higher the aluminum concentration in the body the more the effect happens, resulting in a decreased sperm count and lesser sperm mobility.

# Conclusion, Depopulation and the End Game

In addition to the devastating effect of aluminum on sperm, fetal tissue readily absorbs aluminum just as it does with mercury. So, it seems that aluminum contributes to decreased reproduction in men and women. Adding to this problem is the fact that breast milk contains aluminum in accordance with the aluminum burden in the mother, meaning the more aluminum burden for the mother the more aluminum in the breast milk.

Moreover, infant formulas contain aluminum in significant amounts to be considered contaminated. According to Dr. Chris Exley, baby milk formulas contain so much aluminum because they come in contact with aluminum processing machines and possibly the baby formulas are made from contaminated water. Aside from this, whey protein isolates also contain significant amounts of aluminum.

Right now, in the US, about 45% of all children are suffering from a debilitating disease. Aluminum adjuvants are given to babies at the rate of five at once. Force vaccination is criminal and always a threat. Proper information on the types and effectiveness of vaccines should be provided to all parents so that they can make a proper choice for the health of their child.

About 50% of children diagnosed with autism have problems with intestinal permeability. Like mercury, aluminum accumulates in the gut, it is a sink for heavy metals and often associated with fungal overgrowth, like what typically happens with candida. Without the proper knowledge and guidance on avoiding aluminum and detoxing form it, these kids are destined to be part of the high rates of neuro degenerative disease that keeps affecting younger and younger populations.

An aluminum detox agenda is composed of any easy solution, consume orthosilicic acid in water and food. The only viable sources of orthosilicic acid are in certain waters, vegetables and some grains. In addition, it seems that consuming more vegetables in the diet has the advantages of increasing glutathione and antioxidants as there are more of these in plant matter which also in turn upregulate glutathione production in your genes. Do I recommend you turn into a hardcore vegan? No, we are omnivores by our very nature. However, some people are going to be able to thrive more on different diet combinations, so do your homework and figure out what is best for you. No matter what, it is wise to avoid GMOs, high oxalate foods, processed foods and increase the intake of organic vegetables. Try growing your own.

Regardless as to whether you choose to ignore the evidence for aluminum toxicity or perhaps the controversial chemtrails are too much for you or you flat out disagree with it, aluminum still comes from many other sources that are high enough in concentration to kill you in the long run. This heavy metal causes multiple chronic diseases in the human body. In any case, the end result for the human race on the planet earth is unlikely to be positive, in regards to aluminum toxicity. Remember

## Conclusion, Depopulation and the End Game

that you always have the power to disagree and make your own decisions and this is your right. Choice is always available to you if you choose to acknowledge it. Industry will follow your dollars, so spend them wisely. May the force be with you.

Dr. Bill McGraw, 12-August-21

## Sources and Further Reading

Aluminum Found In Sunscreen: Could It Cause Skin Cancer? https://www.sciencedaily.com/releases/2007/08/070812084458.htm

Aluminum in Daily Life, A Health Risk? https://www.youtube.com/watch?v=ad1L38ST0mA

Atikur Rahman et al. 2018. Importance of Mineral Nutrition for Mitigating Aluminum Toxicity in Plants on Acidic Soils: Current Status and Opportunities. Int J Mol Sci. 2018 Oct; 19(10): 3073.

Auon, A. et al. 2018. The Fluoride Debate: The Pros and Cons of Fluoridation. Prev Nutr Food Sci. 2018 Sep; 23(3): 171–180.

Buettner, D., et al. 2016. Blue Zones, Lessons from the Longest Lived. Am J Lifestyle Med. 2016 Sep-Oct; 10(5): 318–321.

Crouse, K. 2018. Silica Water the Secret of Healthy Blue Zone Longevity in the Aluminum Age. Collins Publishing. USA.

Cutler, A. 1999. Amalgam Illness, Diagnosis and Treatment. Andrew Hall Cutler Books.

Drago, D. et al. 2008. Aluminum Modulates Effects of βAmyloid$_{1-42}$ on Neuronal Calcium Homeostasis and

## Sources and Further Reading

Mitochondria Functioning and Is Altered in a Triple Transgenic Mouse Model of Alzheimer's Disease. Rejuvenation ResearchVol. 11, No. 5. Rejuvenation Research (liebertpub.com)

Ehgartner, Bert. 2018. The Age of Aluminum, Ennstahler Publishing. UK

Exley, Chris.2020. Imagine You Are An Aluminum Atom. Skyhorse Publishing. UK

Feng Ma, J. 1997. Detoxifying aluminium with buckwheat. Nature. volume 390, pages569–570.

Feng Ma, J. 1997. High Aluminum Resistance in Buckwheat: II. Oxalic Acid Detoxifies Aluminum Internally. JSTOR.https://www.jstor.org/stable/4278333.

Flagg, E. et al., 1994. Dietary glutathione intake in humans and the relationship between intake and plasma total glutathione level. Nutrition and Cancer ;21(1):33-46.

Greger.J. 1992. Dietary and other sources of aluminium intake. Ciba Found Symp. 169:26-35

Griffin, G. 1997. World Without Cancer. American Media

Harry Robberecht, Kristien VanDyck, Douwina Bosscher & Rudy Van. 1998. Silicon in Foods: Content and Bioavailability Cauwenbergh. Food Chemistry. Volume 63, Issue 2, October 1998, Pages 235-239

https://drcherylkasdorf.com/wp-con

## Sources and Further Reading

https://www.webmd.com/diet/foods-high-in-oxalates#1tent/uploads/2015/02/OxalateContent092003.pdf

https://jamanetwork.com/journals/jamainternalmedicine/fullarticle/2768887

https://myersdetox.com/transcript-123-how-oxalates-ruin-your-health-with-dr-william-shaw/

https://nutritionfacts.org/es/2016/05/17/aluminum-levels-in-tea/

https://origins.osu.edu/article/toxic-treatment-fluorides-transformation-industrial-waste-public-health-miracle/page/0/1

https://www.apoe4.info/forums/viewtopic.php?t=4022

https://www.geoengineeringwatch.org/category/health/

https://www.geoengineeringwatch.org/category/health/

https://www.pentair.com/content/pentair/en-us/education-support/water-education-center/learn-about-fluoride.html

https://www.statista.com/statistics/254668/size-of-the-global-antiperspirant-and-deodorant-market/

## Sources and Further Reading

https://www.urologyofva.net/articles/category/healthy-living/3740469/11/13/2019/

J P Müller [1], A Steinegger, C Schlatter. 1993. Contribution of aluminum from packaging materials and cooking utensils to the daily aluminum intake. Z Lebensm Unters Forsch. Oct;197(4):332-41.

Julka, D. R K Vasishta, K D Gill. 1996. Distribution of aluminum in different brain regions and body organs of rat. Biol Trace Elem Res. May;52(2):181-92.

Kathrin Ertl, Walter Goessler .2018.Aluminium in foodstuff and the influence of aluminium foil used for food preparation or short time storage. Food Addit Contam Part B Surveill. Jun;11(2):153-159.

Kauffman, Klauss. 1997. Silica, The Amazing Gel. Alive Books. Canada.

Khan, H. et al. 2012.Evaluation of the Interaction of Aluminium Metal with Glutathione in Human Blood Components. April 2012.Biomedical Research 23(2):237-240

Krista,Jones, CarolineLinhart, CliveHawkins, and Christopher Exley. Urinary Excretion of Aluminium and Silicon in Secondary Progressive Multiple Sclerosis.

EBioMedicine. 2017 Dec; 26: 60–67.Liukkonen-Lilja [1], S

## Sources and Further Reading

Piepponen. 1992. Leaching of aluminium from aluminium dishes and packages. Food Addit Contam. May-Jun 1992;9(3):213

Lynch, Ben. 2018. Dirty Genes. Harper Collins. USA.

Mario Müller et al. 1997. Availability of aluminium from tea and coffee. Zeitschrift für Lebensmitteluntersuchung und -Forschung A volume 205, pages170–173

Mazen, A and Maghraby. 1997.Accumulation of cadmium, lead and strontium, and a role of calcium oxalate in water hyacinth tolerance. Biologia
Plantarum volume 40, pages411–417 (1997)

Mazen, A. 2004. Calcium Oxalate Deposits in Leaves of Corchorus olitorius as Related to Accumulation of Toxic Metals. Russian Journal of Plant Physiology. 51(2):281-285

McGraw, Dr. William. 2019. Mercury the Ultimate Truth and Chronic Disease. McGraw Publishing. Panama

Min Yi[1], Huilan Yi, Honghai Li, Lihua Wu. 2010. Aluminum induces chromosome aberrations, micronuclei, and cell cycle dysfunction in root cells of Vicia faba. Environ Toxicol. 2010 Apr;25(2):124-9.

Mouton, M. et al. 2015. Linking the occurrence of cutaneous opportunistic fungal invaders with elemental concentrations in false killer whale (Pseudorca crassidens) skin. Environ Microbiol Rep.Oct;7(5):728-37.

# Sources and Further Reading

Naseem Ullah. 2011. Effect of aluminium metal on glutathione (GSH) level in plasma and cytosolic fraction of human blood. Pakistan Journal of Pharmaceutical Sciences 24(1):13-8

Robberecht , H.et al. 2008. Silicon in Foods: Content and Bioavailability. . Volume 11, 2008 - Issue 3

Salim M Saiyed [1], Robert A Yokel . 2008. Aluminum bioavailability from basic sodium aluminum phosphate, an approved food additive emulsifying agent, incorporated in cheese. Food Chem Toxicol. Jun; 46(6): 2261–2266.

Sripanyakorn et al. 2009.The comparative absorption of silicon from different foods and food supplements. Br J Nutr. 2009 Sep; 102(6): 825–834.

Sripanyakorn, S. 2004. The silicon content of beer and its bioavailability in healthy volunteers..British Journal Of Nutrition 91(3):403-9.

Thorsten Stahl et al. 2017. Migration of aluminum from food contact materials to food—a health risk for consumers? Environ Sci Eur. 2017; 29(1): 19.

van Hulten, M. 2013.,Aluminium in an ocean general

circulation model compared with the West Atlantic Geotraces cruises. Journal of Marine Systems. Volume 126, October 2013, Pages 3-23Vela, M, R.B.Toma, W.Reiboldt,

## Sources and Further Reading

A. Pierri. 1998. Detection of aluminum residue in fresh and stored canned beer. Food Chemistry. Volume 63, Issue 2, Pages 235-239.

Vignal, C. P Desreumaux, M Body-Malapel. 2016. Gut: An underestimated target organ for Aluminum. Morphologie. Jun;100(329):75-84.

Wang, XD et al. 2019. Analysis of aluminum content in unprocessed grains from different areas of China. Zhonghua Yu Fang Yi Xue Za Zhi.Jun 6;53(6):586-589.

Weidenhamer, J. et al. 2017. Metal exposures from aluminum cookware: An unrecognized public health risk in developing countries. Sci Total Environ. Feb 1;579:805-813.

Wise, J. et al. 2018. A three year study of metal levels in skin biopsies of whales in the Gulf of Mexico after the Deepwater Horizon oil crisis. Comp Biochem Physiol C Toxicol Pharmacol. 2018 Feb;205:15-25.

Wise, J. et al. 2019 Metal Levels in Whales from the Gulf of Maine: A One Environmental Health approach. Chemosphere. 2019 Feb;216:653-660.Xin, P.1997. Xian, P. Wild Soybean Oxalyl-CoA Synthetase Degrades Oxalate and Affects the Tolerance to Cadmium and Aluminum Stresses. Int. J. Mol. Sci. 2020, 21(22), 8869.

Yang, J. et l. 2005. Aluminium resistance requires resistance

## Sources and Further Reading

to acid stress: a case study with spinach that exudes oxalate rapidly when exposed to Al stress. Journal of Experimental Botany, Volume 56, Issue 414, Pages 1197–1203.

Zhonghua yu Fang yi xue za zhi [Chinese Journal of Preventive Medicine], 01 Jun 2019, 53(6):586-58

# Index

**INDEX**

***A***

acid reflux · 5, 27

Acidic rainfall · 10

acidic soils · 11, 13, 25

adjuvant · 5

agriculture · 10, 11, 48

**Air** · 16

aluminum foil · 5, 21

aluminum oxides · 48

Aluminum salts · 23, 26

aluminum sulfate · 3, 5, 20, 23, 33

Aluminum sulfate · 20

Alzheimer's · 3, 5, 3, 4, 5, 6, 18, 27, 30, 31, 32, 33, 34, 41, 42, 43, 45, 47, 52

amalgam fillings · 4

antacids · 5, 24, 27

antioxidants · 39, 49, 52

antiperspirants · 3, 26, 37

arteries · 9, 47

autism · 18, 29, 30, 52

***B***

B6 · 15, 16

beer · 21, 40, 56

Bees · 16

black tea · 22

blue zoners · 3, 43

bones · 9, 35, 41, 45, 47

brain · 4, 6, 15, 18, 25, 27, 30, 31, 32, 33, 34, 37, 41, 45, 47, 50, 55

# Index

Brazil · 8

Buckwheat · 23, 54

## C

Calcium · 11, 53, 55

calcium fluoride · 8

calcium oxalate · 12, 14

California · 6, 8, 19

*Cancer* · 2, 6, 51, 53, 54

chemtrail · 5, 17

chemtrails · 5

Chemtrails · 5, 16, 17

China · 8, 52, 57

chlorella · 39

Corn · 23, 47

Crouse · 44

Cutler · 4

## D

Dane Wigington · 17

dementia · 2

depression · 18

Dirty Genes · 49

Dr Ben Lynch · 49

Dr. Chris Shade · 39

dried milk · 3

drugs · 2

## E

e-cigarettes · 3

Environment · 8, 21

Exley · 28, 35, 42, 45, 51, 55

## F

Fluoride · 2, 8, 53

food · 3, 6, 8, 9, 14, 21, 22,

# Index

23, 24, 25, 27, 31, 21, 47, 51, 52, 55, 56

Food · 22, 24, 40, 53, 54, 55, 56

fungi · 13

fungicides · 25

---

**G**

gastrointestinal tract · 39

geoengineeringwatch.org · 17, 18, 50, 54

glutathione · 39, 49, 50, 51, 52, 54, 56

Glutathione · 3, 51, 55

glyphosate · 18, 25

Glyphosate · 18, 25

GMOs · 52

grains · 22, 46, 52, 57

Grains · 23

green beans · 21

Green beans · 21

---

**H**

Hall-Heroult · 9

Heavy metal · 6

heavy metals · 2, 4, 8, 10, 12, 13, 14, 16, 31, 32, 31, 34, 35, 36, 37, 39, 42, 49, 50, 51, 52

herbs · 24, 54

hip fractures · 9, 45

hippocampus · 18, 34

hydroxyaliminumsilicate · 48

hydroxyaluminumsilicate · 11, 12, 42

---

**I**

inflammation · 9, 13, 14, 15, 16, 30, 32, 49

# Index

ionic foot baths · 49, 50

Ionic Foot Baths · 49

iron · 9, 15, 25, 31, 48

## K

kidney stones · 14, 31, 42

Klinghardt · 18, 50

## M

magnesium · 4

Mangel · 19

mercury · 4, 8, 9, 10, 29, 31, 32, 35, 39, 40, 42, 49, 50, 51, 52

milk · 22, 23, 43, 51

Mineral deficiencies · 25

minerals · 4, 9, 10, 11, 13, 31, 37, 45, 47, 48

## N

Nano sized · 18

neuro degenerative · 5, 31, 32, 52

Norton · 15

## O

ocean · 9, 56

orthosilicic acid · 6, 21, 33, 40, 42, 45, 21, 46, 52

OSA · 3, 6, 13, 20, 33, 34, 40, 41, 42, 43, 44, 45, 21, 46, 47

oxalate · 11, 12, 13, 14, 15, 16, 25, 55, 57

Oxalate · 2, 11, 55, 57

oxalates · 12, 13, 14, 15, 16, 25, 54

Oxalates · 2, 12, 13, 14, 15, 16

## P

pancake mixes · 3, 23

# Index

**P**

pH · 2, 8, 10, 11, 13, 25, 41, 48

phosphate · 8, 13, 27, 32, 56

phytolith · 6, 48

phytoliths · 12, 46

pizza · 23

Plants · 12

plastic filling · 4

potassium · 4, 15

pots and pans · 5

pretzels · 23

**R**

rabbit holes · 5

**S**

Selenium · 10

silica · 6, 8, 9, 11, 12, 13, 33, 34, 40, 41, 42, 43, 45, 21, 46, 47, 48, 49

Silica · 2, 11, 41, 44, 47, 48, 49

silicates · 42, 48

sodium silicate · 41, 47oil · 2, 11, 12, 13, 19, 21, 45, 46, 48

soils · 6

soybeans · 23, 25, 48

sperm · 51

spices · 24

spinach · 15, 57

spirulina · 39

sweating. · 14

**T**

Tea · 21, 24

The Dimming · 17

# Index

## V

vaccinated · 2

vaccines · 3

vegetables · 13, 34, 46, 48, 49, 51, 52

viruses · 5, 30, 31

vitamin C · 15, 37, 39

## W

whales · 10, 57

Wi-Fi · 50

## Z

zinc · 10, 35

www.ingramcontent.com/pod-product-compliance
Lightning Source LLC
Chambersburg PA
CBHW052331220526
45472CB00001B/370